Drugs in Breast Milk

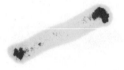

Drugs in Breast Milk

John T. Wilson

 ADIS Press Australasia Pty Ltd
New York · Tokyo · Mexico · Sydney · Auckland · Hong Kong

Drugs in Breast Milk

National Library of Australia
Cataloguing-in-Publication entry

Drugs in Breast Milk

Index
Bibliography
ISBN 0-909337-34-9

1. Milk, human — Contamination
2. Drugs — Physiological effect
I. Wilson, John T., Ed.

612'.664

First printing
ISBN 0-909337-34-9

ADIS Press Australasia Pty Ltd
404 Sydney Road, Balgowlah, NSW 2093, Australia

Preface

Both physicians and the lay public raise questions about drug excretion in breast milk. Enhanced interest is seen with the increase in the number of mothers who wish to breast feed. 'Contamination' of breast milk by drugs and environmental chemicals imposes risks, both known and theoretical, to the infant. Drug information centres and physicians find a meagre amount of knowledge on which to base recommendations and the data which are available are often anecdotal or derived from single case reports. A critical look at both the nature and scope of our knowledge on this matter was undertaken for this review. This purpose was best served by the cooperation of pharmacologists and clinicians who have a special interest in certain classes of drugs. A unified pharmacokinetic approach was formulated to facilitate the evaluation of previous data and to offer a model for future studies.

This work was, in part, published in Clinical Pharmacokinetics Vol. 5 No. 1 1980. Its reception prompted this revised and expanded version and it is hoped that its critical analyses and comprehensive literature citations will foster more concerted and thorough research into drug excretion in breast milk; benefits would then accrue to both maternal and child health.

This work is dedicated to Dr William A. Silverman with whom I was most fortunate to share experiences as a fellow in neonatology and whose dedication to paediatrics and clinical investigation in subsequent years, I have watched from afar. His philosophical abhorrence of data gathering without attention to a hypothesis is particularly germane in this time of technological feasibilities.

We thank Mrs Janis Doyle for her skilful compilation of the manuscript drafts — overstatement cannot adequately describe her dedication. I appreciate the support of my clinical pharmacology research programme given by the Pharmaceutical Manufacturers' Association Foundation. This has enabled the preparation of this review which serves my own research interests and, I trust, those of others.

John T. Wilson
Louisiana State University Medical Center
Louisiana, USA

* Contributors

R. Don Brown, Ph.D.
Professor, Department of Pharmacology and Therapeutics.

D.R. Cherek, Ph.D.
Assistant Professor, Department of Psychiatry, Department of Pharmacology and
    Therapeutics.

John W. Dailey, Ph.D.
Associate Professor, Department of Pharmacology and Therapeutics.

Bettina C. Hilman, M.D.
Professor, Department of Pediatrics; Chief, Pulmonary Allergy Section.

Phillip C. Jobe, Ph.D.
Professor, Department of Pharmacology and Therapeutics; Department of
    Psychiatry.

Barbara R. Manno, Ph.D.
Professor, Department of Pharmacology and Therapeutics.

Joseph E. Manno, Ph.D.
Professor, Department of Pharmacology and Therapeutics; Chief, Section of
    Toxicology.

Helmut M. Redetzki, M.D.
Professor and Chairman, Department of Pharmacology and Therapeutics.

John J. Stewart, Ph.D.
Associate Professor, Department of Pharmacology and Therapeutics.

John T. Wilson, M.D.
Professor, Department of Pharmacology and Therapeutics; Department of Pediatrics;
    Chief, Section on Clinical Pharmacology.

   * All of the above are faculty members of Louisiana State University Medical
Center, Shreveport, Louisiana, USA.

Contents

Glossary of Symbols

AUC   Area under the concentration-time curve for drug in a specified fluid

Compart- 1 = central
ments: 2 = interstitial or intracellular
         3 = breast milk

D   Dose of a drug designated maternal (m) or infant (i)

I   Ionised drug

k_{abs} Absorption rate constant

$k_{el\,\beta}$ Rate constant for overall elimination of a drug from the central compartment

k_{el}, k Elimination rate constant for drug in a specified compartment

M/P   Milk to plasma ratio for drug concentration in each fluid

N   Number of repetitive events

pH $\log \dfrac{1}{[H^+]}$ or $pKa + \log \dfrac{\text{ionised acid}}{\text{un-ionised acid}}$

pKa $- \log k_a$ where k_a = thermodynamic equilibrium acidity constant; pKa is also defined as that pH producing equal portions of the drug in the ionised and un-ionised fraction

t   Time, usually a dosing interval or other specified period; t_B = duration of breast feeding; t_i = interval between breast feedings

$t_{1/2\,abs}$ Half-life for absorption

$t_{1/2\,\beta}$ Half-life for β-phase elimination of a drug from the central compartment

U   Un-ionised drug

V   Volume of designated fluid

Vd   Apparent volume of distribution for a drug in the body or in a specified compartment

1

An Information Gap

John T. Wilson

The perspicacious pen of Lewis Thomas (1979) captures both the purpose of this monograph and our apprehension about the information gap in the field of drug excretion in human breast milk:

' . . . *It is this sudden confrontation with the depth and scope of ignorance that represents the most significant contribution of twentieth-century science to the human intellect.*'

The excretion of drugs in breast milk has been reviewed previously (Anderson, 1979; Shirkey, 1980; Catz and Giacoia, 1972; Hervada et al., 1978; Knowles, 1965, 1972, 1973, 1974; Vorherr, 1974). These reviews emphasise that most data about the presence of a drug in human breast milk are available from single case reports. Mechanistic concepts about drug excretion in milk have been developed from animal studies. A rational basis is needed for extrapolation of these data to man. Pharmacokinetics operative for a particular drug need to be developed in cognisance of fundamental processes for breast milk excretion. The paediatric consequences of drug dosing via breast milk also need attention if the matter is to be placed in perspective. In this monograph multiple aspects of the excretion of drugs in breast milk are reviewed and an unfortunate lack of human pharmacokinetic data on medicines and chemicals likely to be consumed during lactation highlighted.

2

Prevalence and Advantages of Breast Feeding

John T. Wilson

An estimated 96% of mothers are able to breast feed under favourable conditions (Sedgwick, 1921) and when feeding techniques are known (Applebaum, 1975; Blaikley et al., 1953; Waller, 1946). In the United States, the number of mothers who breast feed at the time of hospital discharge has been increasing: 25% in 1974 (Fomon, 1974), 38% in 1975 (AAP, 1978) and 53% in 1976 (AAP, 1978). These figures compare with 35% in Canada (AAP, 1978) and 70% in Sweden (Vahlqvist, 1975) for the mid-1970's. The incidence falls to 5% by 6 months postpartum for women in all of these countries.

Breast milk is the only food the infant needs for the first 4 to 6 months of life although some supplementation with vitamin D and fluoride is advised (AAP, 1978). Phylogenetic differences in suckling (and milk composition) are presupposed adaptations to immaturity of the organism at birth (Bostock, 1962; Jelliffe, 1969). The scope of these differences is illustrated by the very immature offspring of the platypus (ova) and kangaroo (fetus) or the more mature human (exterogestate of 9 months) and sea lion (transitional). Relative immaturity of each species determines the duration of breast feeding. The continuous contact nature of human suckling also serves to keep prolactin levels high and to delay sequential pregnancy. Additional advantages and rationale for breast milk feeding are shown in table I. Further appreciation of these matters will increase the prevalence of breast feeding in the future as well as strengthen compliance with feeding routines needed for pharmacokinetic investigations.

Table I. Advantages of breast feeding and breast milk[1]

Maternal
1. Maternal bonding
2. Less cost than substitute products
3. More appropriate child spacing due to a decrease in fertility
4. Portable and resists spoilage while in the breast

Infant
1. Infant bonding
2. Decreased incidence of diarrhoea, wheezy bronchitis, necrotising enterocolitis
3. Bactericidal effect of lysozyme
4. Presence of C_3 and C_4 components of complement, lactoferrin, secretory IgA and small amounts of IgM and IgG
5. Lower morbidity in first year of life
6. Bifidus factor stimulates growth of *L. bifidus* in gut
7. Iron better absorbed and less anaemia found
8. Lower incidence of tetany due to Ca/P ratio
9. Less obesity and less chance of marasmus
10. More digestible
11. Decrease in food allergy (compared with cow's milk which has high β-lactoglobulin)
12. Composition tailored to organ development (e.g. renal function) and growth (e.g. term compared with premature infant).

---

1 Data from Klaus et al. (1970); Klaus and Kennell (1976); Lynch (1975); Kolodny et al. (1972); American Academy of Pediatrics (1978); Barness (1977); Jelliffe and Jelliffe (1978); Taitz (1975); Cunningham (1977); Foman (1974); American Academy of Pediatrics (1976); Atkinson et al. (1978).

It has been stated that use of milk substitutes is one of the largest uncontrolled experiments performed in man (Hambraeus, 1977). The long term consequences of a lack of breast feeding, as compared with those of feeding breast milk containing drugs and other chemicals, is cause for concern and immediate study.

3

Production and Characteristics of Breast Milk

John T. Wilson

1. Mammary Gland Structure and Permeability

The breast contains specialised mammary glands which evolved from and are morphogenetically similar to sweat glands. Each breast contains 15 to 25 lobes (glands) which are subdivided into lobules. Functional units can be described as a 'mammon' composed of secretory cells surrounding a lumen (alveolus), ducts, and blood supply. Alveoli are connected by larger ducts which empty into collecting or lactiferous ducts. These ducts have a dilation (sinus lactiferous) prior to their termination in the nipple. The luminal or duct contents are separated from the extracellular space by a biological 'membrane' composed of basement membrane, myoepithelial cells, and low columnar glandular cells. A network of blood vessels surrounds the alveolus on its basal lamina surface. Vascular innervation is noradrenergic. Secretory cells and myoepithelial cells have no nerve supply.

Although some preformed, endogenous, systemic substances are found in milk (Rasmussen, 1973), a selective blood-milk barrier exists for the mammary ducts of most species studied. In the goat, no bidirectional transfer of sodium, rubidium, or chloride could be shown (Linzell and Peaker, 1971b). The duct membrane is permeable to water, but milk remains isosmotic to plasma. The secretory cell of the alveolus is rich in storage granules (lactose and protein), fat globules, and in endoplasmic reticulum near the basal portion of the cell.

Table II. Hormonal control of breast milk production[1]

Origin	Hormone[2]	Effects
Prepartum		
Placenta	Oestrogens and progesterone	Hypothalamus: inhibits prolactin release through an inhibition factor (PIF)
		Adenohypophysis: induction of prolactin synthesis
		Breast: duct, lobular and alveolar development; some milk synthesis begins with aid of supportive metabolic hormones[3]
Postpartum		
Hypothalamus	PIF decreased PRF increased	Adenohypophysis synthesis and release of prolactin
Adenohypophysis	Prolactin	Breast milk synthesis and letdown reflex[3]
Neurohypophysis	Oxytocin	Breast: milk ejection reflex

1 See also Vorherr (1972).
2 PIF = Prolactin inhibiting factor; PRF = Prolactin releasing factor.
3 Supportive hormones include growth hormone, parathyroid hormone, thyroid hormone, cortisol, insulin.

2. Secretion of Breast Milk

A merocrine secretory process is responsible for protein and water secretion in breast milk. This process yields little contamination from cytoplasm of mammary alveolar cells. Apocrine (tip of apical cell is shed) and holocrine (whole cell is shed) processes also contribute to milk production but to a lesser extent (Linzell and Peaker, 1971b). The apocrine process is used for fat secretion.

Breast milk secretion is under hormonal control (table II) and offers many possibilities for enhancement or inhibition by drugs. Oestrogen and progesterone have a facilitatory role, but high progesterone can inhibit differentiation of breast tissue and milk secretion. The increase in prolactin levels after delivery promotes synthesis and secretion of milk. These follow in reflex manner from an increase in sucking (Jelliffe and Jelliffe, 1978). High prolactin levels in serum are found with prolonged sucking (Nichols and Nichols, 1979). Prolactin secretion is susceptible to drug modification. It is decreased by levodopa, ergocriptine and bromocriptine and increased by phenothiazines, amphetamine, methyldopa and theophylline (Kulski et al., 1978; Vorherr, 1974a,b). Growth hormone, ACTH, insulin, cortisol, thyroid hormone, and parathormone are required for optimum milk secretion and yield (Catz and Giacola, 1972; Linzell and Peaker, 1971c; Reynolds, 1969; Rivera and Bern, 1961). Selective but sequential roles for insulin, hydrocortisone, and prolactin have been

Table III. Exogenous influences on breast milk production[1]

Maternal
1. Subcutaneous fat gain during pregnancy (affects energy for lactation and is sensitive to nutritional state)
2. Undernutrition, fad diet or inadequate diet, slimming diet postpartum, restrictive food customs
3. Timing of meals, especially in relation to fat content of milk
4. Psychosocial stress (inhibits early more than established lactation)
5. Sequential reproduction and prolonged lactation (debilitates the mother)
6. Hard work or, conversely, physiological restrictions leading to less energy use
7. Menses
8. Conditioning (e.g. wet nurses who have a large volume of milk)
9. Drugs — inhibition by oral contraceptives

Infant
1. Sucking — amount, vigour and frequency
2. Body weight
3. Number of offspring
4. Behaviour (reinforces psychosocial bonding and allays stress of breast feeding)
5. Unknown (note that kangaroo can secrete milk of different composition from each teat to meet developmental needs of the young)

1   Data from Jelliffe and Jelliffe (1977, 1978); Hytten and Leitch (1971); Nims et al. (1932a,b); Wichelow (1976).

defined in cultures of mammary gland explant in regard to epithelial cell division, endoplasmic reticulum proliferation, Golgi complex enlargement, and the complete differentiation of the cell for synthesis of casein and lactose (Mills and Topper, 1970; Turkington et al., 1971). Oxytocin is released from the posterior pituitary in response to sucking. This hormone causes contraction of myoepithelial cells around alveoli to express milk into ducts (the 'milk ejection' or 'draught reflex'). Oxytocin release is especially sensitive to inhibition by anxiety or lack of confidence for breast feeding (Vorherr, 1974a).

Other maternal and infant factors influence the production of milk (table III) and hence the amount of drug available from this route.

3. Blood Flow and Milk Production

Lactation is associated with a high blood flow to the breasts, gut and liver as well as an increase in cardiac output (Hanwell and Linzell, 1973; Peaker, 1976; Pickles, 1953). Blood flow to the breast is 400 to 500-fold greater than the volume of milk produced (Linzell, 1974). Mammary vessels are very sensitive to vasoconstrictors, so that blood flow is decreased by sympathetic stimulation (Linzell, 1950; Peeters et al., 1949), adrenaline (Hebb and Linzell, 1951), stress (Linzell, 1960), and fasting

(Linzell, 1967). Stress effects on blood flow are independent of an action on the milk ejection reflex (Hanwell and Linzell, 1972; Linzell, 1974) since such effects are mediated by noradrenergic innervation of mammary vessels. Altered blood flow during menstruation decreases milk production.

4. Volume (yield) and Water Content of Milk

Early data on milk yield was misleading because samples were collected from conditioned wet nurses (Nims et al., 1932a,b) and arbitrary volumes were calculated to meet caloric requirements of the infant. Daily volumes from Swedish women were similar for the years 1945 (Walgren, 1945) and 1975 (Lonnerdal et al., 1976a): 558

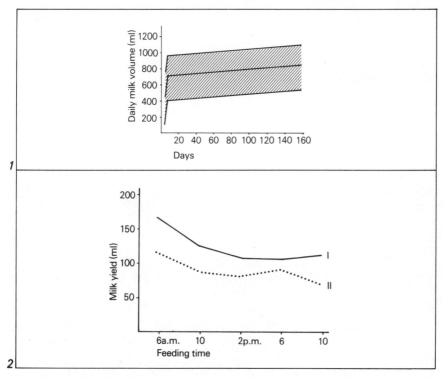

Fig. 1. Total daily milk volume produced by well nourished Swedish mothers. Solid line in the middle of the striped area = regression line for the 50 mothers. Striped area = tolerance interval to this regression line (Lonnerdal et al., 1976b).

Fig. 2. Mean diurnal variation in the yield of milk. Curve I represents milk from the 21st day of lactation or later. Curve II represents earlier milk (Hytten, 1954).

to 611ml at 1 month, 752 to 766ml at 3 months and 756 to 779ml at 6 months. A more recent Swedish study (Svanberg et al., 1977) showed a mean of 838ml/day. The United States mean for daily yield of breast milk is somewhat lower: 606ml at 1 month, 601ml at 2 months and 625ml at 3 months (Jelliffe and Jelliffe, 1978).

All studies emphasise a marked intersubject variation in yield (e.g. at 3 months, the daily range was 400 to 900ml). This is emphasised by figure 1 which also shows that a high rate of milk secretion is not seen until 3 to 4 days. It rises to a plateau by about 1 month and is sustained for 6 months in Western cultures (Lonnerdal et al., 1976b; Peaker, 1976). For a given individual, the volume varies each day and a diurnal pattern is seen. A maximum yield occurs at 6am and a nadir at 6pm or 10pm (Hytten, 1954; Jelliffe and Jelliffe, 1978) [fig. 2].

Influences on yield include the stress of hospitalisation (Lindblad et al., 1976), infant size and sucking pattern, and twin as compared with single infant nursing (Addy, 1975; table III). Undernutrition decreases milk yield, even to the point of infant starvation, under extreme conditions of food deprivation (Jelliffe and Jelliffe, 1971; Waletzky and Herman, 1976). Diet supplements can correct a nutritional basis for decreased yield (Deb and Cama, 1962). Approximately 30 calories from the diet are needed to produce 20 calories in milk (Nichols and Nichols, 1979). Yield is directly related to blood flow and prolactin secretion (Linzell, 1974). For each feeding,

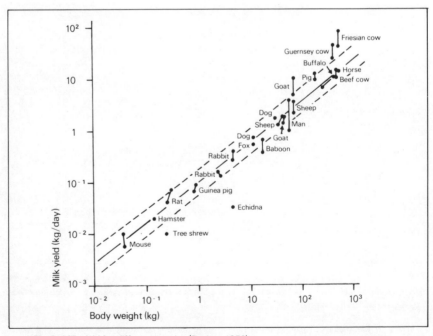

Fig. 3. Milk yield for different species (Peaker, 1976).

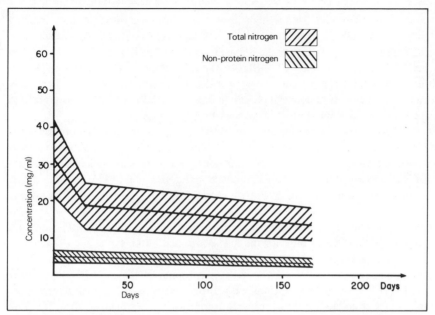

Fig. 4. Concentrations of total nitrogen and non-protein nitrogen in breast milk from well nourished Swedish mothers. Protein = total nitrogen less non-protein nitrogen (redrawn from Lonnerdal et al., 1977).

the yield from each breast is not similar but depends on how well it was emptied during the previous feeding (Hytten, 1954). A correlation exists between size of species and daily volume of milk (fig. 3) [Peaker, 1976]. The technique of milk collection must be standardised if accurate inter-study comparisons of milk yield are to be made (Hytten, 1954).

Water comprises the major part of milk (87 to 95 %) [Jelliffe and Jelliffe, 1978; Peaker, 1976] and it is not influenced by amount of water consumed. A net increase in water turnover occurs with some coming from intake and some from renal conservation (antidiuretic effect of prolactin). In the alveolar cell, lactose draws water into the Golgi apparatus to help form the aqueous phase of milk (Linzell and Peaker, 1971a,b,c). Ducts in different parts of the mammon are permeable to water, but milk remains isosmotic with plasma since lactose, the primary osmol, is not reabsorbed during active lactation.

5. Protein Content and Composition of Milk

Protein content of milk is 0.8 to 0.9 % according to recent estimates made by amino acid analysis (Lonnerdal et al., 1976a,b). An increased capillary permeability is considered responsible for the high protein concentration in colostrum compared with mature milk. Protein (total nitrogen less non-protein nitrogen) falls rapidly during the first week postpartum and a more gradual decline is seen after 20 days (Hytten, 1954; Lonnerdal et al., 1977) [fig. 4]. Mature milk shows little diurnal or feed-to-feed variation in protein content (Hytten, 1954; Jelliffe and Jelliffe, 1978). Hind milk contains 1.5-fold the amount of protein in fore milk (Hall, 1975) and it is postulated that this results from water displacement by fat (Hytten, 1954).

There is no evidence for an influence of age or parity on protein content, but variable data are obtained when lactation is continued into the second year postpartum (Jelliffe and Jelliffe, 1978). Malnutrition or even supplementation of the maternal diet does not affect daily protein production (Edozien et al., 1976; Gopalan, 1958; Gopalan and Belavady, 1961; Jelliffe and Jelliffe, 1978; Lindblad and Rahimtoola, 1974). Some interindividual variation is seen (about 20%; see fig. 4). Protein concentration is higher in milk secreted for premature infants and the rate of postpartum decline parallels that of milk for the full term infant (Atkinson et al., 1978).

Precipitation of casein produces a whey protein which is 60 to 70% of total protein in human milk (Bell and McKenzie, 1964; Hambraeus et al., 1976; Lonnerdal et al., 1977). Casein contains calcium and phosphorus and shows species differences in the curd due to amino acid composition (Hambraeus, 1977). The methionine/cysteine ratio approximates 1.0 and there is a low content of alanine and tyrosine. The β, κ and α_{S1} caseins predominate in breast milk (Jelliffe and Jelliffe, 1977a,b,c). The major whey proteins in man are α-lactalbumin, lactoferrin, secretory IgA, serum albumin and lysozyme (Lonnerdal et al., 1977). β-Lactoglobulin predominates in cow's milk (Bell and McKenzie, 1964).

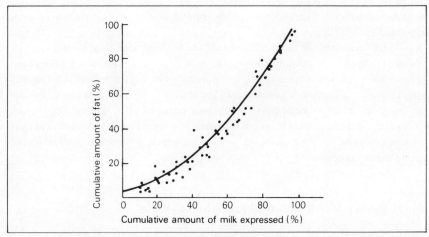

Fig. 5. Relation between fat content and milk yield. Twelve fractionated samples were analysed from 3 subjects milked to complete expression (Emery et al., 1978).

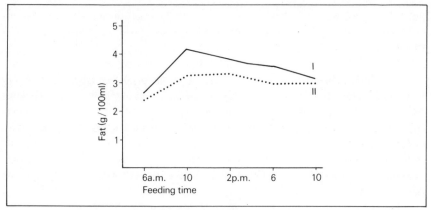

Fig. 6. Mean diurnal variation in the fat content of milk. Curve I represents milk from the 21st day of lactation or later. Curve II represents earlier milk (Hytten, 1954).

Secretory IgA is present in concentrations of 4 to 5mg/ml colostrum and 1 to 3mg/ml mature milk (Lonnerdal et al., 1977). It is distinct from that in serum and is acid pH-resistant (Hambraeus, 1977). Marked interindividual variation is seen for milk content of α-lactalbumin and lactoferrin (Lonnerdal et al., 1976a,b). The average concentration of α-lactalbumin is 163 ± 6mg/100ml (Hartmann and Kulski, 1978). Immunoglobulin IgG and IgM are also found, the highest levels being in colostrum.

Human milk contains more taurine and cysteine and less tyrosine and phenylalanine (Jelliffe and Jelliffe, 1977a,b,c; Sturman et al., 1970) than does cow's milk. Enzymes are associated predominantly with membranes or cellular debris in milk. A lipoprotein lipase is present but milk does not contain a lactase (Nichols and Nichols, 1979). Human breast milk contains about 25% of nonprotein nitrogen (e.g. urea, creatine, creatinine, uric acid, small peptides and free amino acids) compared with about 5% in cow's milk (Hambraeus, 1977).

6. Fat Content and Composition of Milk

Fat is the primary source in milk and the average content is 2.1 to 3.3% (Foman, 1974; Hytten, 1954, Morrison, 1952). Fat content is increased by an uninhibited letdown reflex (Hall, 1975) and decreased by malnutrition (often as low as < 1%). Hind milk contains 4 to 5-fold the amount of fat in fore milk and this is maintained for 3 to 35 weeks postpartum (Hall, 1975). An increased rate of fat production in milk is seen during the last half of feeding from a breast (Emery et al., 1978) [fig. 5]. This is thought to be due to fat absorption to alveoli and ducts. The terminal steep slope for fat content versus feeding time is presumably related to a prolonged sojourn for fat in the breast (Hytten, 1954). Additionally, the milk ejection reflex forces more fat from the secretory cell into the ducts during a feeding period (Nichols and Nichols, 1979). A similar pattern is seen in cows (Johannson et al., 1952).

The rate of rise in fat content of milk is different for each breast. A higher initial level in fore milk is seen with higher residue from the prior feed (Hytten, 1954) or when short intervals prevail between feedings (Evans and MacKeith, 1958; Hytten, 1954; Kon and Mawson, 1950). A diurnal variation in fat concentration is found (Hytten, 1954) [fig. 6]. These factors obviate a single milk collection as representative of the 24-hour mean for fat content (Hytten, 1954) or for amount of substances excreted in breast milk fat. Rapid estimation of fat content is obtained from 'creamatocrits' (normal range 1 to 9 %), which correlate well with total fat and calories in breast milk (Lucas et al., 1978).

The composition of milk fat is affected by the maternal diet. A recent 2-fold increase in milk linoleic acid is probably secondary to the increase in dietary vegetable fat and polyunsaturated fats (Guthrie et al., 1977; Widdowson et al., 1974). Fatty acid content does not change from fore to hind milk (Emery et al., 1978). A high carbohydrate diet increases the content of saturated fatty acids in milk (Insull et al., 1959; Read et al., 1965) whereas a decreased caloric intake yields a fatty acid profile similar to that in maternal subcutaneous deposits (Cuthbertson, 1976; Insull et al., 1959; Welby et al., 1973). Cholesterol is higher in hind milk and in colostrum (Picciano, 1978; Potter and Nestel, 1976; Tarjan et al., 1965). Total lipid increases and the profile of fatty acids changes from a 12 to 14 carbon species as colostrum progresses to mature milk (Read and Sarrif, 1965). Triglycerides comprise 81 % of the lipid content of human milk (Nichols and Nichols, 1979),

7. Lactose Content of Milk

Mature human milk contains 6.9 to 7.2 % lactose (Morrison, 1952; Kon and Mawson, 1950) and it is not affected by undernutrition (Jelliffe and Jelliffe, 1978). Fore and hind milk content is similar (Hall, 1975), although some decrease is seen as fat increases (Hytten, 1954). A systematic pattern of diurnal variation in lactose content is not found and there is an irregular difference in content from feed to feed (Hytten, 1954). Lactose is synthesised *in situ* and does not back diffuse from milk. It is the primary osmol and 'traps' water (Linzell and Peaker, 1971a,b,c). The specifier enzyme for lactose synthesis is α-lactalbumin and it is extruded into milk with lactose (Brew, 1969; Brodbeck and Ebner, 1966; Brodbeck et al., 1967; Keenan et al., 1970; Watkins and Hassid, 1962).

8. Ionic Composition and pH of Milk

Compared with other species, human milk is low in sodium and potassium, presumably due to its lactose content which serves to maintain isotonicity with

Table IV. Composition of milks obtained from different mammals (adapted from Hambraeus, 1977; Hollman, 1974)

Species	Content of milk (%)					Diameter of protein granules (A)
	water	fat	protein	lactose	ash	
Man	88.1	3.8	0.9	7.0	0.2	300
Horse	88.9	1.9	2.5	6.2	0.5	
Cow	87.4	3.7	3.4	4.8	0.7	800-1200
Reindeer		16.9	11.5	2.8		
Goat	87.7	4.5	2.9	4.1	0.8	
Sheep	81.3	7.4	5.5	4.8	1.0	
Rat	68.0	15.0	12.0	3.0	2.0	1500-3000

Adapted from Hambraeus L: Proprietary milk versus human milk in infant feeding, Pediatric Clinics of North America 24: 17-26, 1977, and Hollman, K.H.: Cytology and fine structure of the mammary gland, in Larson, B.L. and Smith, V.R. (Eds): I. The Mammary Gland/Development and Maintenance, Academic Press, Inc., New York and London, 1974.

regard to plasma (Peaker, 1976). Milk has a positive potential when compared with the intracellular milieu which its K/Na ratio resembles (Peaker, 1976). The basal (but not apical) portion of the secretory cell has a Na-K pump and is inhibited by ouabain (Linzell and Peaker, 1971a). The Na and K content of milk is established by an energy-requiring process which can be influenced by blood flow (Linzell and Peaker, 1971c). Phosphorus content is about one-seventh of cow's milk, and calcium is one-third, probably as a result of low casein in human milk. The content of iron is less than in cow's milk (Picciano and Guthrie, 1976), whereas zinc levels are comparable (Eckert et al., 1977). Iodide is concentrated in milk by an uptake system similar to that in the thyroid, as noted from the effect of perchlorate and thiocyanate on the mammary gland in animals (Brown-Grant, 1957; Reineke, 1961). It should be recalled that a selective blood-milk barrier for the reabsorption of Na, Rb, Cl ions in the ducts has been described for the goat (Linzell and Peaker, 1971a,b).

Very few studies have reported the pH of human milk under conditions known to influence volume or composition. One study (Hall, 1975) reported the following rise in pH in fore to hind milk: 7.2 at 2 minutes, 7.3 at 5 minutes, and 7.4 at 15 minutes; buffering capacity did not change during this time. Others cite a pH 7.0 or a range of 6.35 to 7.65 (average 7.08) for human milk (Rasmussen, 1973; Yurchak and Jusko, 1976). These pH values indicate a species difference when compared with cow's and goat's milk which has a pH of 6.6 to 6.8 (Rasmussen, 1973). Such differences affect prediction of drug excretion in breast milk.

9. Feeding Pattern and General Data Relevant to Pharmacokinetic Studies

The infant pattern of feeding influences both the dose of milk and of drug content. About half the volume, protein, lipid and energy are taken in the first 5 minutes of sucking. In the last 11 to 16 minutes, the infant consumes 13% of total volume, 16% of protein and energy, but 25% of fat (Hall, 1975). The post-feed residual in the breast is estimated at 52ml (Hall, 1975). The infant's decision to stop feeding on one breast and move to the other may be a function of taste, smell and/or texture of milk (Evans and MacKeith, 1958; Hall, 1975). The dictum of 10 minutes of feeding on each breast is artificial. Milk produced between feedings remains in the alveoli and minor ducts. Oxytocin and the ejection reflex are required to get milk into the lactiferous duct. Prolonged cessation of feeding promotes regressive changes in glandular epithelium and affect both the accumulation and reabsorption of milk.

Each breast has its own fore to hind cycle, and milk composition during a feeding is not the same in each, although the tendency is towards similarity (Barrie et al., 1975; Hytten, 1954). This confounds interindividual variation in rate and extent of changes in breast milk composition (Hall, 1975; Hytten, 1954). These caveats apply to milk sample collection and milking devices [Humalactor breast pump (Hytten, 1954)] if representative and 'natural' pharmacokinetic data are to be obtained.

Species differences in suckling pattern, milk volume, and composition (table IV) clearly identify the human lactating female as the only suitable model for drug excretion studies designed to predict the amount of drug consumed by the infant.

4

Pharmacokinetics of Drug Excretion

John T. Wilson

Since human breast milk is an aqueous fluid of heterogeneous and varying composition, the amount of drug excreted in milk will vary with both the composition and yield. Fundamental processes for xenobiotic elimination (i.e. transport and metabolism) determine which drugs will be excreted. Physicochemical properties of the drug (or its metabolite) influence both its passage and 'trapping' into milk components. Maternal dose and compliance are the important determinants of the drug dose delivered to an infant by a regular schedule of breast feeding.

The complex nature of drug dosing via breast milk is summarised by a list of factors as described in table V. An accurate approach to both excretion rate and concentration of a drug in breast milk depends on integration of all pertinent pharmacokinetic factors. For this purpose, an understanding of each factor and its susceptibility to maternal, drug, or infant influences, is needed. Knowledge is primarily derived from animal studies although restricted sampling in women has provided some data on milk (M) to plasma (P) drug concentration ratios. The following discussion will emphasise human data and animal to man extrapolations where feasible so that fundamental pharmacokinetic principles can be derived.

1. Blood Flow

While blood flow increases during lactation (see section 3.3), little is known about flow during or between feedings. General estimates have been made in cows

Table V. Factors affecting excretion of a drug in breast milk and dose consumed by infant

---

1. *Maternal Pharmacology*
   a) Drug dose, frequency and route
   b) Clearance rate
   c) Plasma protein binding
   d) Metabolite profile

2. *Breast*
   a) Blood flow and pH
   b) Yield capacity
   c) Ion and other transport mechanisms
   d) Drug metabolism (and reabsorption?)

3. *Milk*
   a) Composition (fat, protein, water)
   b) pH

4. *Infant*
   a) Suckling behaviour, including equal time on each breast
   b) Amount consumed per feeding
   c) Feeding intervals (regular or irregular)
   d) Time of feeding in relation to maternal dosing

5. *Drug*
   a) pKa (ionisation at plasma and milk pH)
   b) Solubility characteristics in fat and water
   c) Protein binding characteristics
   d) Molecular weight

---

and goats by the use of antipyrine and the Fick principle (Rasmussen, 1963, 1965; Rasmussen and Linzell, 1964; Reynolds et al., 1968). A high residue of milk impedes blood flow to mammary tissue and decreases milk yield. Similar effects are seen with vasoconstrictive agents. High mammary blood flow during the time of peak drug absorption would be expected to deliver a greater quantity of drug to milk. Studies have not been undertaken to determine whether the breast exhibits high or low clearance properties for certain drugs in a manner similar to that described for the liver. Nevertheless, it is important to assess the relationship of flow changes with breast feeding so that the drug administration schedule will administer the smallest possible amount of drug to the infant.

2. Protein Binding

The extent and affinity of drug binding to both plasma and milk proteins are a determinant of drug concentration in whole milk. This is of special note since alveolar

Table VI. Comparison of drug binding in milk and plasma from cows and goats[1]

Drug	% Bound[2]		Factor[3]
	milk	plasma	
Pentobarbitone	40-50	72-68[a,b]	0.6
Phenobarbitone	29-45	70-80[b]	0.5
Salicylic acid	32	75[a]	0.4
Benzoic acid	15	42[a]	0.4
Para aminohippurate	5	29[a]	0.2
Antipyrine	0	0[a]	1
Ephedrine	0	0[a]	1

1 Data are calculated from results of Miller et al. (1967a,c).
2 % bound estimated by:

$$\frac{\text{total concentration} - \text{ultrafiltrate concentration}}{\text{total concentration}} \times 100$$

3 Factor = Binding in milk compared with that in plasma.
a Cow
b Goat

cells apparently do not have many active transport systems for 'stripping' drugs from plasma proteins. A lower M/P concentration ratio for whole milk was found for several sulphonamides, as the percentage of plasma protein binding increased from 8 to 50%. A higher plasma as compared with milk protein binding was associated with a M/P concentration ratio of less than 1. The ultrafiltrate M/P ratio was higher than that for whole milk when plasma binding was higher than that of milk (Rasmussen, 1971). The situation for these drugs can be depicted diagrammatically as in figure 7.

Binding of some drugs in milk was found to be generally lower than that for plasma (table VI). For cows and goats, bound drug in milk was 0.2 to 0.6% that of plasma. Neither the degree nor affinity for drug binding have been assessed for the milk-specific proteins. For example, is the drug binding shown in table VI predominantly a function of casein, α-lactalbumin, or other milk proteins? Species and individual differences in protein concentration are expected to produce differences in binding and hence total drug excreted in milk. The role of competing drugs and endogenous ligans for binding sites has not been determined.

3. Ionisation

The degree of drug ionisation, and hence the availability of un-ionised drug to traverse the lipid biological membrane, has been extensively studied in cows and goats. Approaches are based primarily on two rearrangements of the Henderson-Hasselbach equation (Davson and Danielli, 1943; Jacobs, 1940; Rasmussen, 1973) to provide the following % of un-ionised drug:

Acid $\log \dfrac{U}{I} = pKa - pH$ (Eq. 1)

Base $\log \dfrac{I}{U} = pKa - pH$ (Eq. 2)

where U and I = concentration of un-ionised and ionised drug, respectively, and pKa = drug pKa; pH = pH of fluid in question. (Note that U + I = total drug concentration in the ultrafiltrate).

The ratio of total drug in an ultrafiltrate of milk compared with plasma (M.ult./P.ult. ratio) is:

Acid M.ult./P.ult. $= \dfrac{1 + 10^{(pHm - pKa)}}{1 + 10^{(pHb - pKa)}}$ (Eq. 3)

Base M.ult./P.ult. $= \dfrac{1 + 10^{(pKa - pHm)}}{1 + 10^{(pKa - pHb)}}$ (Eq. 4)

where pHm = pH of milk; pHb = pH of blood.

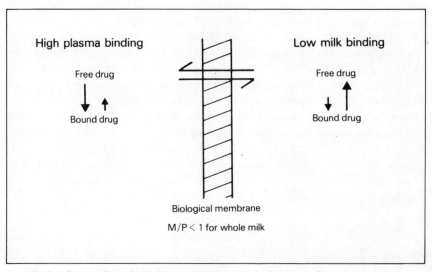

Fig. 7. Influence of protein binding on drug concentration in breast milk.

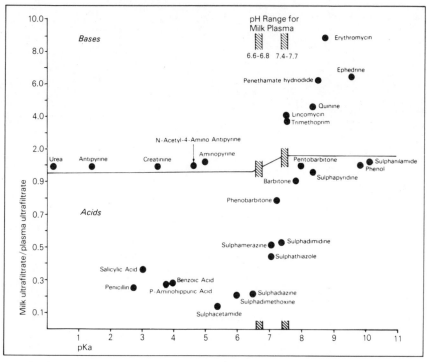

Fig. 8. Ratio of the ultrafiltrate drug concentration for milk and plasma of cows and goats. A plot of experimental M/P ultrafiltrate values for various drugs was made from data of Rasmussen (1971).

Prerequisites to utilisation of ion-partitioning concepts for drug distribution are:

1) Drug pKa and fluid pH are the only determinants of distribution
2) Ratio is independent of fluid volume of the compartment
3) The un-ionised drug is soluble in the lipid phase
4) Ratio is applicable to only the free fraction of the drug
5) Ratio is independent of the plasma drug concentration (Miller et al., 1967c).

Certain generalisations have emerged from animal studies to support the conclusion that the un-ionised portion of free drug diffuses across the lipid biological membrane (Brodie, 1964; Bodie and Hogben, 1957; Schanker, 1962, 1971) into milk such that an equilibrium is established between this portion in the aqueous phase of milk and plasma at a given plasma concentration of a drug. The concentration of un-ionised drug (antipyrine, sulphadimidine and trimethoprim) was found to be similar in milk and plasma and hence the ultrafiltrate M/P ratio for un-ionised drug approached unity, even though disparate pKa's and a different percentage of un-ionised fraction as compared with total drug was found (Rasmussen, 1973).

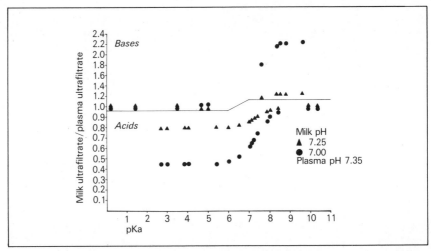

Fig. 9. Estimated M/P ratio for a drug in ultrafiltrate of human milk and plasma. The M/P ultrafiltrate ratio was estimated for those drugs shown in figure 8 according to their pKa values as reported by Rasmussen (1971).

In general, the ultrafiltrate M/P ratio for weak acids is <1 and for bases is >1. This has been shown for sulfadoxine and penicillin (Rasmussen, 1958, 1966, 1973) and for trimethoprim and erythromycin (Rasmussen, 1959, 1973). The relationship between ionisation and pH was established for pH 6.8 to 8.1 by injection of bicarbonate into the cow udder (Miller, 1967c). The M/P ratio for un-ionised drug in milk or plasma ultrafiltrate did not change concomitantly with a change in milk pH (6.9 to 7.3, 7.6 and 6.4), while a steady-state plasma concentration of sulphadiazine was maintained by infusion (Rasmussen, 1959, 1971). The ionised portion of a drug in milk or plasma would be expected to change as pH varied during normal breast feeding in man (Hall, 1975) and hence drug 'trapping' in milk would occur.

Species differences in plasma and milk pH between animals as compared with man will alter the amount of free drug distributed in the ultrafiltrate. A pH 6.6 to 6.8 and 7.4 to 7.7 is found for cow or goat milk and plasma respectively (Rasmussen, 1971, 1973). Some drug M/P ratios for the ultrafiltrate fractions show close agreement between observed and theoretical values predicted from the pKa. A plot of the M/P ratio relationship with pKa is seen in figure 8. Acids with a high pKa (e.g. phenol, sulphanilamide) and bases with a low pKa (e.g. antipyrine, creatinine) do not show much change in the M/P ultrafiltrate ratio at pH 6.6 to 8.1 (Miller et al., 1967a,b) as expected. Urea remains 100% un-ionised and its distribution is little affected by changes in milk pH. In contrast to cows and goats, the milk of lactating women shows an average pH of 7.0 (Rasmussen, 1973; Vorherr, 1974a) or 7.25 (Hall, 1975). Recalculation of the M/P ultrafiltrate ratio for drugs shown in figure 8 and in regard to human milk pH reveals the same general pattern (fig. 9). However, the M/P ratio for a weak acid or base is quite different, depending on the pH of milk (compare pH 7.0 to 7.25). The influence of ionisation on the M/P ratio diminishes as the pH difference narrows. Cross-species comparisons of drug concentrations in milk ultrafiltrates can be misleading if the pH characteristics of the fluids are not considered.

4. Lipid Solubility

The coefficient of lipid solubility for an un-ionised drug determines both its penetration of the biological membrane to gain entrance to milk and also its concentration in milk fat. Drug partitioning into lipids of different composition has not been studied, but is of conceivable importance, given the variability in both composition and content of milk lipids (see section 3.6). Even though a drug may be 100% un-ionised, if its lipid solubility is low (e.g. urea), then absorption through a lipid membrane will be slow (Rasmussen, 1971). Sulphonamides with low fat solubility are found primarily in the aqueous and protein fraction of milk whereas many barbiturates appear in the lipid fraction (Rasmussen, 1958, 1966, 1973). Levels of salicylic acid in plasma equilibrated faster with milk than did those of p-aminohippuric acid (Miller et al., 1967c). An inverse relationship between concentration of drug in skim milk and its coefficient of lipid solubility is shown in figure 10. This relation-

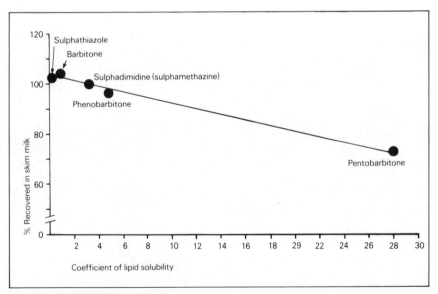

Fig. 10. Relationship between lipid solubility and recovery of a drug in skim milk. Data reported by Rasmussen (1971) are plotted.

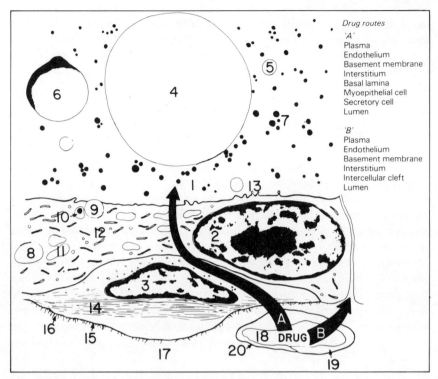

Fig. 11. Transit path of a drug from blood to milk.

Diagrammatic sketch adapted from an electron photomicrograph of mouse mammary tissue (Rhodin, 1977).

1) Lumen of alveolus.
2) Nucleus of secretory epithelial cell.
3) Nucleus of myoepithelial cell.
4) Large milk lipid droplet suspended in luminal fluid.
5) Small milk lipid droplet.
6) Lipid droplet retaining detached peripheral coat of cytoplasm.
7) Milk protein particles.
8) Lipid droplet in cell cytoplasm.
9) Lipid droplet near cell surface.
10) Protein particle in a vacuole.
11) Mitochondrion.
12) Short profiles of granular endoplasmic reticulum.
13) Short microvilli.
14) Bundle of myofilaments.
15) Basal lamina.
16) Reticular fibrils.
17) Loose connective tissue.
18) Lumen of blood capillary.
19) Endothelium.
20) Basal lamina of capillary.

ship demonstrates the importance of knowing the fat content of milk in order to estimate drug content in whole milk.

5. Transfer Processes (diffusion, transport)

Egress of a drug from the capillary lumen occurs by diffusion or reverse pinocytosis. In the mammary interstitial space the drug exists in several states: ionised, un-ionised, protein-bound or bound to cell membrane. Permeation of the mammary epithelium occurs primarily by diffusion of the un-ionised species of the drug. Transport by the action of carrier and lipophilic proteins is an additional minor mechanism. Active transport has been found for very few drugs. Ionised and/or small molecular weight xenobiotics (MW < 200) penetrate water filled pores in the membrane. Exit from the alveolar cell occurs by apical diffusion, apocrine secretion or through membrane pores (Singer, 1973; Vorherr, 1974a).

A drug passes through multiple structures to gain entry to milk by 1 of 2 routes (fig. 11). In route A, the drug moves through multiple membranes and intracellular fluids to finally emerge in the alveolar lumen. Transit through membranes is via the lipid portion (for un-ionised drugs with high lipid solubility) or via water filled pores surrounded by protein 'icebergs' (for water-soluble, presumably low molecular weight drugs) [Singer, 1973]. In route B, a drug enters milk more directly by way of an intercellular cleft. Route preference for certain drugs is not known. Route A offers an opportunity for drug binding or metabolism by the alveolar cell.

Evidence is convincing for the primary role of diffusion of an un-ionised drug from blood and interstitial fluid into breast milk. Observed and predicted values for the ultrafiltrate M/P drug concentration ratio show close agreement when the degree of ionisation is considered. Un-ionised drug concentration shows similar values for milk and plasma while total drug in the ultrafiltrate changes with alteration in pH. This relationship for most un-ionised drugs is not changed at different plasma levels (Rasmussen, 1971, 1973).

Active secretion of a drug into milk has been described in animals for aminopyrine (Banerjee et al., 1967), N^4-acetylated para aminohippuric acid (Rasmussen, 1969a), and N^4-acetylated sulphanilamide (Rasmussen, 1969b). As the plasma concentration of acetylated PAH rose in cows and goats, the M/P ratio for total drug decreased from 4.1 to 0.8. This is consistent with an active but saturable transport process (Rasmussen, 1969a,b).

6. Metabolism

Once inside the alveolar cell a drug may be metabolised prior to exit. This has been shown for sulphanilamide which is N^4-acetylated by mammary tissue

(Rasmussen and Linzell, 1967). The finding of microsomes in breast milk (Morton, 1953) raises the unlikely possibility of drug metabolism in milk. It should be noted that finding drug metabolites in milk is not necessarily evidence for their formation by mammary tissue. Metabolites of diazepam (Erkkola and Kanto, 1972), chloramphenicol (Vorherr, 1974a) and isoniazid (Berlin and Lee, 1979) have been found to be excreted into milk from plasma.

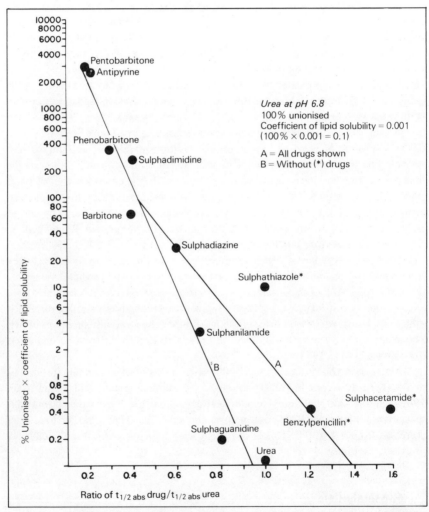

Fig. 12. Relationship of drug lipid solubility and un-ionised fraction at pH 6.8 to reabsorption rate in breast milk as compared with that for urea. Data reported by Rasmussen (1971) are plotted. The reason for divergence of drugs marked with (*) on line A is not known.

7. Excretion into Alveolar Lumen

Drug in the alveolar cell may be expelled into the milk-containing lumen by diffusion or concomitantly with secretion of fat droplets and protein granules. Additional studies are needed to investigate the role of concomitant secretion as a means of drug entry into milk.

8. Reabsorption

Drug reabsorption from human breast milk has not been confirmed but is central to the design of pharmacokinetic approaches and to estimates of the amount of drug delivered to the infant via breast milk. As noted in sections 3.7 and 3.8, reabsorption of lactose and certain ions in cow's milk does not occur. However, evidence from retrograde injection studies in cows and goats strongly implicates drug reabsorption in these species. An exponential decay from udder to venous blood has been found for sulphacetamide and sulphanilamide (Rasmussen, 1971) and for potassium chloride (Knutsson, 1964; Knutsson and Sperber, 1964). A $t_{1/2\ abs}$ for drug absorption from the udder could be calculated by:

$$t_{1/2\ abs} = \frac{2.303 \times \log 0.5}{-\lambda} \qquad \text{(Eq. 5)}$$

where λ = slope of the decay curve. The relationship of $t_{1/2\ abs}$ of these sulphonamides to that of urea and for different milk pH's indicated that reabsorption was by diffusion of un-ionised drug. A high lipid solubility promoted a short $t_{1/2\ abs}$. The relationship of ionisation and lipid solubility to drug reabsorption as compared with urea reabsorption is shown in figure 12.

Evidence for drug absorption in man comes from a few studies of concomitant decay of drug concentration in plasma and milk (Yurchak and Jusko, 1976). Studies of a drug distributed in aqueous medium (e.g. antipyrine) need to be made at frequent intervals by taking a small sample from one breast while the other is completely milked. Comparable concentrations and decay characteristics for milk from both breasts would indicate drug reabsorption. This approach is depicted in figure 13 which also shows a comparison with plasma concentrations following administration of a drug dose. It is apparent that the derived data would allow milk to plasma comparisons of AUC, $K_{el\ \beta}$, $t_{1/2\beta}$ and Vd. An estimate of drug concentrations in milk could be made for selected times after a dose. These estimates could then be compared with observed concentrations during breast feeding (see section 4.10).

9. Volume of Milk

Rapid bidirectional diffusion of a drug between plasma and milk obviates concentration differences secondary to milk yield changes in cows and goats (Rasmussen,

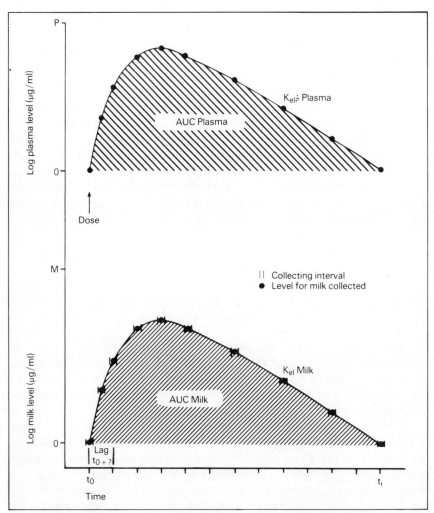

Fig. 13. Plasma drug concentration and decay kinetics compared with those in milk. An idealised relationship is shown for drug concentrations in milk (M) compared concomitantly with those in plasma (P). A lag period, if it exists, is shown as t_0 + ? (an unknown period of time). The decay profile is depicted for a t_i corresponding to a customary interval (about 6 hours) between breast feedings and for a drug with a $t_{1/2} \simeq 3$ hours (i.e. so that a significant decay occurs during the feeding interval). Drug in milk profile is represented as being the same for both breasts.

1958, 1961, 1966). Repeated milking with a small yield produced the same concentration of sulphathiazole as a single milking with large yield. Similar results have been obtained for antipyrine, ethanol, urea (Rasmussen, 1961), iodide (Miller and Swanson, 1963) and barbiturates (Rasmussen, 1966). A similar situation in man would simplify pharmacokinetic correlates for drug concentration in plasma and milk and for timing of feedings in relation to dosing.

10. An Integrated Approach to Pharmacokinetic Investigation

The variable nature of milk secretion and composition as well as the multiple influences on drug excretion in milk warrant the design of an integrated approach. This or other suitable approaches can be used for analysis of data presented in subsequent sections and to highlight more specifically the need for additional studies.

Breast feeding in relation to drug dosing and steady-state plasma concentrations for a typical day is shown in figure 14. Breast feeding occurs at different times in rela-

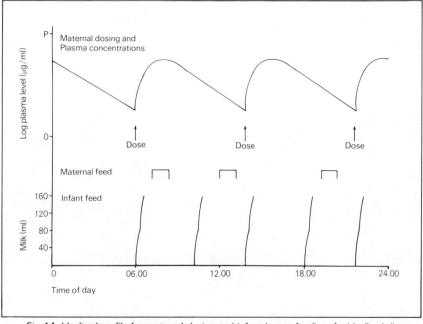

Fig. 14. Idealised profile for maternal dosing and infant breast feeding. An idealised diagram for breast feeding and dosing is shown. The milk volume plot represents the known rapid secretion of fluid during the early period of breast feeding. The 'notch' in the plot depicts a change from one breast to the other. Plasma concentrations are shown for steady-state conditions and the drug is assumed to have a $t_{1/2} \simeq 3$ hours for reasons cited in figure 13.

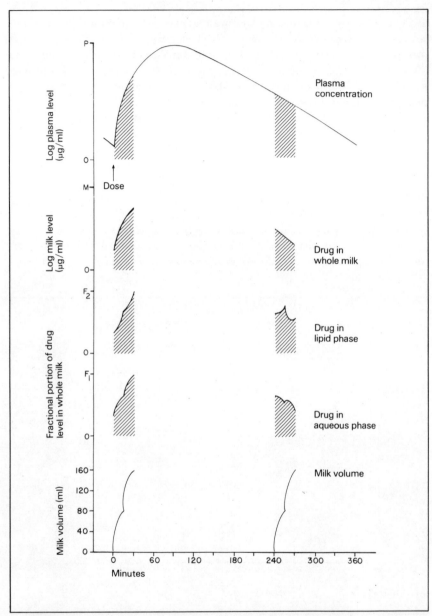

Fig. 15. Pharmacokinetic relationships between milk and plasma drug levels for 2 breast feedings during a dosing interval. See legends for figures 13 and 14. The fractional portion of drug concentrations in the aqueous and lipid phases shows differences during the suckling period in accordance with the rate of excretion of each phase. The infant suckled for about 15 minutes on each
breast.

tion to dose and hence drug concentrations in milk will vary according to some relationship with plasma concentrations.

As seen in figure 15, frequent and concomitant measurements of drug concentration in milk and plasma can be made during breast feedings which occur at different times in relation to a dosing interval. These measurements provide meaningful data for calculation of the M/P ratio and for assessment of average concentrations during a feeding. For these purposes, the following expressions are used:

$$M/P = \frac{AUC_3}{AUC_1} \qquad\qquad (Eq.\ 6)$$

where 3 and 1 refer to milk and plasma, respectively.

$$Average\ conc. = \frac{AUC_3}{t} \qquad\qquad (Eq.\ 7)$$

where t is the interval for AUC estimation.

Predictions of drug excretion in milk can be made if the pKa and lipid solubility coefficient of the drug and protein binding, protein and fat content and pH are known for both plasma and milk. The influence of each variable can be assessed as additional measurements are made daily and on subsequent days. Drug concentrations in aqueous or lipid fractions of whole milk can be estimated to test these predictions (fig. 15). An average of milk composition and drug AUC analysis over a period of several days will give a more accurate estimate of drug excretion in breast milk. Maternal plasma drug levels must be assessed for steady-state conditions to make meaningful predictions of dose delivered to the infant during protracted dosing of the mother. Several plasma or urine samples from the infant can be analysed to substantiate projected exposure from breast milk dosing.

11. Calculation of Dose Received by the Nursing Infant

The approaches described above are useful for the calculation of the average amount of drug delivered to the infant during breast feeding:

$$Dose = \frac{AUC_3}{tB} \cdot V_{3,tB} \qquad\qquad (Eq.\ 8)$$

where tB = period of time for breast feeding; AUC_3 is the area under the curve for drug concentration (mg/L) in milk during tB; and V_3, tB is the volume of milk consumed during t_B. The daily dose (D) is calculated by:

$$Dose \times N_B = Dose/day \qquad\qquad (Eq.\ 9)$$

where N_B = number of breast feedings per day. The body weight adjusted dose is:

Daily dose/infant body weight (kg) = Dose/kg/day   (Eq. 10)

This can then be compared with the recommended dose for an infant to assess the relative exposure. The amount of drug recovered in the infant's urine can be used to assess the accuracy of dose calculations or to estimate the amount of drug absorbed by the infant.

A known Vd and $t_{1/2}$ for the drug in infants can be used to estimate the plasma concentration at steady-state ($\overline{C}_{pss}$) [Wagner et al., 1969] where the infant dosing interval (t) corresponds to the interval between breast feedings and the dose to the infant (D_i) is the amount of drug delivered via breast milk:

$$\overline{C}_{pss} = \frac{D_i}{Vd \cdot k_{el\beta} \cdot t}$$ (Eq. 11)

$$\left(\text{note that } k_{el\beta} = k_{10} = \frac{0.693}{t_{1/2\beta}} \right)$$

For this example, 100% bioavailability is assumed. Analysis of an infant plasma sample collected at a time corresponding to 5 to 7 half-lives after onset of breast feeding will evaluate the accuracy of the prediction and allow comparison with known therapeutic or toxic concentration for the drug.

A more precise approach to estimate the dose from drug concentrations in milk (C_3) at a given time would be to use the integrated expression:

$$C_{3,t} = C_{3,0} e^{-k_{el_3}t}$$ (Eq. 12)

where $C_{3,0}$ is the initial concentration; k_{el3} is the overall rate constant for drug elimination from milk (probably equivalent to $k_{el\beta}$ for the central compartment under a normal routine of breast feeding); and t is the time from $t_0 \rightarrow tB$ [i.e. the time from onset (t_0) to termination (tB) of breast feeding]. If breast feeding occurs during the absorption phase then both k_{abs} (absorption rate constant) and k_{el3} must be used to calculate $C'_{3,t}$:

$$C'_{3,t} = \frac{M}{P} \cdot \frac{D}{Vd} \cdot \frac{k_{abs}}{k_{abs} - k_{el}} (e^{-k_{el_3}t} - e^{-k_{abs}t})$$ (Eq. 13)

where M/P is used to adjust the difference between drug concentration in milk and that in plasma. The above expression is for calculation of $C'_{3,t}$, which is the milk concentration at time t after a single maternal dose. The $C'_{3,t}$ after repetitive dosing could be calculated by adding $C_{3,0}e^{-k_{el_3}t}$ to the above expression. When $t = t_0$, then $C_{3,0}$ is the milk concentration of drug just prior to the subsequent dose. For these calculations, it must be assumed that no lag exists between time to peak concentration for plasma and milk, or that k_{abs} can be determined for milk rather than plasma samples.

The following summation for each $C_{3,t}$ would give the total dose delivered in milk during the period of breast feeding:

$$\sum_{t_0}^{t_B} C_3 = \text{Amount of drug/total milk vol.} = D_i = \qquad\qquad \text{(Eq. 14)}$$
$$C_{3,t_1} \cdot V_{3,t_1} + C_{3,t_2} \cdot V_{3,t_2} + C_{3,t_n} \cdot V_{3,t_n}$$

where N is the number of time intervals chosen under the condition that $V_{3,tB}$ is not exceeded and where each V_3 as indicated is the volume of milk analysed for the concentration $C'_{3,t}$ expressed in units per ml. In general, the precision offered by this approach has little practical value since the period of breast feeding represents a small segment of the $t_{1/2}$ for most drugs (fig. 15). The approach is more important for pharmacokinetic modelling and predictions of dose or concentration in milk at a selected time after onset of a breast feeding.

12. Pharmacokinetic Model of Drug Disposition in Breast Feeding

We propose that drug concentrations in breast milk exhibit kinetic decay characteristics of a deep compartment. This concept is shown digrammatically in figure 16. Infant modulation of the amount of drug in the deep compartment is an important feature of this model. The 'rate constant', k_{30}, approximates zero order during

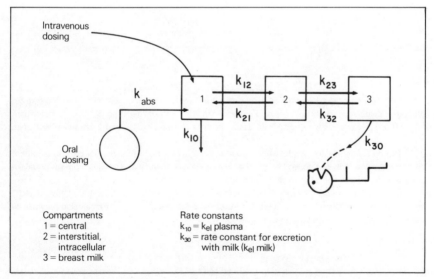

Fig. 16. An infant-modulated 3-compartment open model for drug excretion in breast milk.

feeding but the actual rate fluctuates according to the infant sucking pattern. With lack of nursing, $k_{30} = 0$ and this allows accumulation of milk and drug in the third compartment. This drug is available for transfer to compartment 2 (assuming that drug absorption from milk occurs in lactating women). It is presumed that k_{21} is higher than that for the deep compartment (k_{32}), and thus k_{32} would be rate-limiting for drug elimination from compartment 1 when:

$$k_{32}Vd_3C_3 > k_{10}Vd_1C_1 \qquad\qquad \text{(Eq. 15)}$$

where C_3 and C_1 represent concentration of drug and Vd_3 and Vd_1 represent the volume of drug distribution in the third and first compartments, respectively. The rate of elimination of drug from compartment 1 reflects the rate from compartment 3 when the amount of drug in the latter becomes substantial. This condition should prevail when breast milk engorgement occurs following cessation of nursing for a prolonged period, concomitant with a prolonged interval subsequent to a drug dose.

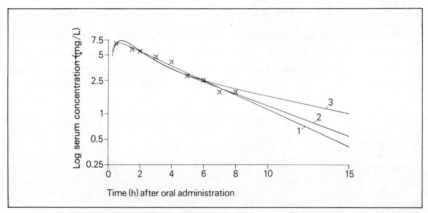

Fig. 17. Proposed plasma decay profile of a drug sequestered in breast milk. The drug is given orally and disposition as shown by plot 3 is according to the model depicted in figure 16 but where $k_{30} = 0$. Plots 1 and 2 are derived from assumption of a respective 1- and 2-compartment open model.

The decay profile for all plots (to 6 hours) is calculated from theophylline data in a patient described by Yurchak and Jusko (1976). The γ decay profile (plot 3) is *projected* from an apparent change in terminal slope of drug disappearance from milk in the same patients.

Data are not sufficient beyond 6 hours to confirm a γ decay for plot 3. Note that plots 2 and 3 are simultaneous through 5 hours. The hypothetical rate constants (α,β,γ) were calculated by use of the ESTRIP programme (Brown and Manno, 1978).

Compartments	α	β	γ	r^2
1		0.199976		0.99
2	1.03524	0.1646		0.97
3	2.64918	0.66077	0.0941	0.998

r^2 = squared correlation coefficient of estimates made by ESTRIP.

A 3-compartment, open, mammillary model with breastmilk being a compartment attached to the central compartment could also exist. Dimensions of k_{13} and k_{31} would more directly determine temporal aspects of the milk to plasma drug concentration profile. For this model it is assumed that k_{12} and k_{21} are greater than k_{13} and k_{31}. It is also probable that $k_{31} > k_{13}$. Sufficient differences must exist in the rate constants to distinguish those for drug transfer between the central compartment and the second or third compartment. Drug disposition measured in plasma of the pre- and post-lactating woman is one approach to assess magnitude of rate constants concerned with drug excretion in milk. Monitoring of drug accumulation and elimination in plasma and milk after a dose (fig. 13) can also be used.

Results from several studies support either of the proposed 3-compartment open models. The time to absorption peak shows a plasma to milk lag in breast feeding women treated with carbamazepine (Blacker et al., 1962), ethanol (Kesaniemi, 1974), theobromine (Resman et al., 1977) and theophylline (Yurchak and Jusko, 1976). [See also that for captopril on p. 64]. An apparent decreased terminal elimination rate for drug in milk as compared with plasma was found for theophylline in lactating women (Yurchak and Jusko, 1976) and for nortriptyline and amitriptyline in lactating rabbits (Jorgensen, 1977).*

A prolonged terminal or a gamma (γ) phase of plasma drug elimination would be apparent when a large amount of milk accumulates in the gland as occurs with decreased emptying of breasts between feedings. This phase would be especially evident for a drug with a short $t_{1/2 \, \beta}$ (fig. 17), or for a compound with $M/P \gg 1$.

Drug elimination rates in non-lactating women may not be applicable to nursing mothers if large amounts of drug exist in a deep compartment represented by a breast engorged with milk. Existence of this compartment would thus present a unique situation with regard to drug disposition. It 'opens' only during lactation, and drug egress is by 2 routes, excretion (k_{30}) and back diffusion (k_{32}). The depth and capacity of this postulated third compartment in the model remain to be assessed. However, a compartment described as deep and of moderate to limited capacity would appear most likely.

Note added in proof: Prolonged sojourn of salicylic acid and morphine in breast milk compared with plasma (Findlay et al., 1980) provide support for the proposed pharmacokinetic model. See also results for salicylic acid reported by Berlin et al., 1980.

5

Analytical Procedures

Joseph E. Manno

The analysis of breast milk for drugs, environmental agents, and other compounds can be readily accomplished by using standard analytical procedures. The primary difference between breast milk and other body fluids normally analysed is that breast milk contains a relatively high concentration of fatty acids and related lipids. These lipid materials can reduce extraction efficiency and also interfere with analyses, particularly gas liquid chromatography. Accordingly, multiple solvent extractions are necessary for the complete extraction of compounds with high lipid solubility. The removal of lipids as a source of interference has been accomplished by several techniques which include washing with a low polarity solvent such as hexane (Baty et al., 1976; Buchanan et al., 1969; Clyde and Shute, 1956; Krzeminski et al., 1972; Pacifici and Placidi, 1977; Sack et al., 1977; Werthmann and Krees, 1972; West et al., 1975), column chromatography (Manes et al., 1972), protein precipitation prior to extraction (Panalaks, 1970), steam distillation (Wiskerchen and Weishaar, 1972), lyophilisation (Mee, 1974), and washing (Kahn and Kerber, 1971).

Horning et al. (1973) studied the recovery of several acidic and basic drugs from breast milk. High recoveries for most drugs (range 84 to 98 %) were observed with ethyl acetate or isopropanol as extractants. Chromatographic interference from lipids was removed by reconstituting the extraction residues with an ethanol-acetic acid-water (8:1:1) solution and washing with hexane. The hexane wash effectively removed lipids but lowered recoveries by about 20 %. The procedure serves as a starting point for development of drug analytical methods.

Table VII. Analytical procedures used for measurement of drugs and other substances in human breast milk

Analytical method	Compound	Reference
Gas-liquid chromatography	Insecticides	Bakken and Seip (1976)
	Vitamin D	Panalaks (1970)
	Nitrofuran	Ryan et al. (1975)
	Chlorobutanol	Wiskerchen and Weishaar (1972)
	Diazepam	Cole and Hailey (1975)
	Methadone	Blinick et al. (1975)
		Kreek et al. (1974)
	Ethanol	Kesaniemi (1974)
	Warfarin	Baty et al. (1976)
		Orme et al. (1977)
	Nicotine	Ferguson et al. (1976)
	Glutethimide	Curry et al. (1971)
	Halothane	Cote et al. (1976)
	Pinazepam	Pacifici and Placidi (1977)
Thin-layer chromatography	Prednisone	Katz and Duncan (1975a,b)
	Vitamin K_1	Manes et al. (1972)
	α-Tocopherols	Herting and Drury (1967)
Atomic absorption spectrophotometry	Metals	Kahn and Kerber (1971)
		Murthy and Rhea (1971)
		Dillon et al. (1974)
Radioimmunoassay	Prolactin	Malven and McMurtry (1974)
	Thyroxine	Sack et al. (1977)
	Norgestrel	Thomas et al. (1977)
High performance liquid chromatography	Theobromine	Resman et al. (1977)
	Theophylline	Yurchak and Jusko (1976)
Spectrophotometry, UV, visible or fluorescence	Chloramphenicol	Havelka et al. (1968)
	Nitrites and nitrates	Wegner (1972)
	Chlorpromazine	Blacker et al. (1962)
	Mefenamic acid	Buchanan et al. (1968)
	Flufenamic acid	Buchanan et al. (1969)
	Pyrimethamine	Clyde and Shute (1956)
Tritium label	Prednisolone	McKenzie et al. (1975)
Enzymatic	Methotrexate	Johns et al. (1972)
Gamma x-ray spectrometry	Gold	Blau (1973)
Electrophoresis	Nitrofurantoin	Varsano et al. (1973)
Gas chromatography-mass spectrometry	Phenobarbitone	Horning et al. (1973)
	Quinalbarbitone (secobarbital)	
	Caffeine	
	Phenytoin	
	Morphine	
	Diazepam	

A wide variety of analytical procedures has been successfully employed for the qualitative and quantitative estimation of drugs and environmental agents in milk (table VII). The analysis of breast milk for additional drugs and other chemicals can be accomplished by utilising methods previously developed for assaying other body fluids. Slight modification of methods may be necessary because of interference from lipids or lack of adequate recoveries.

6

Psychoactive Substances and Antiepileptic Drugs

Phillip C. Jobe

The pharmacokinetics of psychotherapeutic drug passage into breast milk are of special importance since drugs in this class are in wide use by many individuals, including nursing mothers. Drug therapy must often be continued throughout the nursing period for those with epilepsy, severe paranoid schizophrenia, or recurrent endogenous depression and suicidal ideation.

1. Benzodiazepines

Some benzodiazepines are excreted into breast milk when they are administered to lactating mothers. Patrick et al. (1972) found that oxazepam, an active metabolite of diazepam, was present in the urine of an 8-day-old infant, nursing from a mother who had received diazepam (30mg/day) for the previous 3 days. Only a qualitative determination was made. The infant became lethargic and experienced loss of weight within 2 days after the mother began taking diazepam. Electroencephalographic recordings showed EEG bursts of rapid activity in the frontal regions and were consistent with the expected effects of a sedative medication.

Erkkola and Kanto (1972) found that diazepam and another of its active metabolites, N-demethyldiazepam, were both present in the mother's milk and the nursing infant's blood on days 4 and 6 after parturition. Each of the 3 mothers included in the study received diazepam (30mg/day) for 6 days after delivery. As would be expected from the $t_{1/2\beta}$ for diazepam of 2 to 8 days in adults, the concentration of this drug and its demethylated metabolite increased from day 4 through to day 6 in the mother's blood and milk. In contrast, the mean concentration of diazepam and N-demethyldiazepam in the infant's blood on day 6 decreased respectively to less than 43% and 12% of the day 4 mean values. The possibility that these decreases resulted from a reduced milk consumption by the infants appears remote because of the data obtained from weighing each infant before and after feeding. Although 2 of them consumed slightly less milk each day, the third infant maintained a steady intake but still experienced a decrease in benzodiazepine blood levels from days 4 through to 6. As an alternative explanation, the authors suggested that the decrease in plasma drug concentrations was due to a maturation of a drug biotransformation system in the infant.

Another important observation from the study of Erkkola and Kanto (1972) is that the concentrations of diazepam and N-demethyldiazepam in each of the 2 infants' blood were quite high at 4 days, being 172 and 243µg/ml, respectively. At this point, their mean diazepam blood concentration was 35% of that in the mothers', whereas the metabolite level was 71% that of the mothers' blood.

Diazepam concentrations were consistently higher than those of N-demethyldiazepam in maternal and infant blood as well as in milk (Erkkola and Kanto, 1972). These observations of milk concentrations contrast markedly with those of Brandt (1976) who reported N-demethyldiazepam concentrations to be 100 to 150% of diazepam concentrations in the 4 lactating mothers studied who received a dosage of 10mg daily. According to Brandt's observations, this can be explained by the relative degree of binding of diazepam (98%) and N-demethyldiazepam (97%) to plasma proteins. Since 2% of diazepam and 3% of N-demethyldiazepam exist as free drug, it is apparent that the plasma concentrations of the unbound metabolite are 150% of the unbound diazepam. According to Brandt (1976), this is more than enough to allow the concentrations of N-demethyldiazepam to be 100 to 150% of diazepam concentrations in milk. In our view, this argument for an ultrafiltrate of milk is valid as far as it goes. However, it does not address itself to the question of ion trapping differences in plasma concentration of parent drug and metabolite, or protein binding in milk. The concentration ratio of parent drug and metabolite in milk could be reversed by an appropriate shift in their relative degree of protein binding. If the ratio were sufficiently altered, diazepam could predominate in milk, as was observed by Erkkola and Kanto (1972).

Other benzodiazepines such as chlordiazepoxide, oxazepam and clorazepate (a pro-drug for N-demethyldiazepam) are probably excreted in breast milk, but adequate documentation is lacking. O'Brien (1975) recommended that clorazepate not be administered to mothers who are nursing their infants. This was based on the manufacturer's opinion and no supporting data to the contrary are present. The International Drug Therapy Newsletter (Ayd, 1973) claims that chlordiazepoxide and clorazepate are excreted in breast milk and offers a 'personal communication' from Hoffmann-La

Roche, as evidence. The Newsletter further contends that since oxazepam 'is a major metabolite of diazepam, it is quite likely that it would be present in breast milk'. Catz and Giacoia (1972) state that 'chlordiazepoxide is excreted into breast milk in minimal amounts, whereas diazepam does not pass into breast milk'. In support of this statement, they too, offer as evidence a 'personal communication, Roche Laboratories'.

2. Barbiturates

Phenobarbitone (phenobarbital) is present in the breast milk of animals in concentrations sufficient to increase hepatic drug metabolic enzyme activity in nursing progeny (Fouts and Hart, 1965). Fahim and King (1968) found that nursing animals exhibited reduced growth and increased mortality rates when their mothers were given phenobarbitone in doses of 50mg/kg/day. These doses were much larger than those used to produce sedative, anxiolytic, or hypnotic effects in humans. Also, uterine responsiveness to exogenous oestrogen was decreased in the progeny. On the basis of these observations, Fahim and King (1968) suggested that phenobarbitone, obtained from mother's milk, induced alterations in the rates of gonadal steroid metabolism in developing neonates.

Using a qualitative detection procedure, Tyson et al. (1938) reported that phenobarbitone was present in milk of lactating humans taking sedative (30mg 4 times daily) and hypnotic (90mg at bedtime) doses of the drug. The mothers in this study received phenobarbitone from the sixth day after delivery until they were discharged from the hospital (7 to 11 days postpartum). Samples of milk were taken on each of these days. Phenobarbitone was detectable in the milk beginning on the first day of drug administration. In 1 set of 11 mothers receiving hypnotic doses of phenobarbitone, 2 infants reportedly became difficult to awaken and slept excessively.

The death of an infant who nursed from a mother treated with phenobarbitone was reported by Juul (1976). Since this drug was present in detectable amounts (8.3µg/ml) in the infant's blood, phenobarbitone-induced sedation was implicated as a contributing cause of death.

More recent investigations reported by Coradello (1973) show that barbiturates administered in antiepileptic doses (i.e. in amounts of 60 to 200mg/day which typically produce maternal blood concentrations of 10 to 30µg/ml) are not detectable in breast milk. If, as suggested by Vorherr (1974b), phenobarbitone concentrations in milk are 1.5% of those in plasma, the concentrations in milk should not exceed 0.45µg/ml. Even when blood phenobarbitone concentrations are 60µg/ml, the average amount in milk would be only 0.9µg/ml. If an infant consumed 1000ml of milk/day, clinical signs and symptoms of intoxication would not occur except in cases of undue sensitivity to the effects of this drug. [See a recent review by Rane (1978) for a thorough description of barbiturate disposition in the neonate].

Barbiturates other than phenobarbitone are excreted into breast milk (Horning et al., 1975). Butabarbitone (butabarbital) concentrations were reported to be 0.37µg/ml in milk 1.5 hours after the 7th dose in an example where 8mg of the drug was given twice daily to a lactating mother. Pentobarbitone (pentobarbital) levels were 0.17µg/ml 19 hours after the last dose, given to mothers who had received 100mg daily for 3 days. Also, quinalbarbitone (secobarbital) was found in milk 14 hours following the last dose (amount not specified). 14 minutes after completion of an intravenous infusion (1.125g in 35 minutes), the level of thiopentone (thiopental) was 20µg/ml in milk (Mayo and Schlicke, 1942).

3. Central Nervous System Stimulants

Relatively little information is available regarding the passage of many of the CNS stimulants into breast milk. None of the nursing infants, born to 103 lactating mothers treated with amphetamine, showed any detectable behavioural stimulation or insomnia (Ayd, 1973). However, times of administration, ages of mothers or infants, and nursing schedules were not described. The amount of amphetamine which passes into breast milk has not been established because of the difficulty in the solvent extraction techniques (Ayd, 1973). Difficulties with analytical methodology preclude detection of methylphenidate in breast milk.

Caffeine was found in human breast milk following the consumption of tea or coffee (Irvin, 1926; Schilf and Wohinz, 1928; Schumacher, 1936). The mean concentration of caffeine in breast milk was approximately 8.2µg/ml when 6 mothers drank coffee (containing a total of 100mg of caffeine) 4 hours before analysis. About 1% of the caffeine was recovered in approximately 100ml of milk at 4 hours (Schilf and Wohinz, 1928). It is possible that higher concentrations occurred at other time intervals since neither the peak concentration nor the time to peak concentration of caffeine in milk was determined. If the average milk concentration was 8.2µg/ml at each feeding, then the total dose of caffeine for a baby who drank 1 litre of this milk per day would be 8.2mg/day. However, some people consumed much more than 100mg of caffeine within the course of a few minutes. Consequently, the amount in mothers' milk might be several times higher than the predicted 8.2µg/ml.

Recent studies have demonstrated the passage of other methylxanthines such as theobromine and theophylline in human milk (Yurchak and Jusko, 1976; Resman et al., 1977). These are reviewed in section 6.4.5.

4. Marijuana

According to Hervada et al. (1978), there are no reports that Δ^9-tetrahydrocannabinol (THC, the primary active moiety of marijuana) passes into breast milk. He further states that 'a few unconfirmed cases of drowsiness have been reported in nursing infants after their mothers smoked marijuana'. However, no supporting literature citations are offered.

Studies of lactating dams show that THC is excreted in breast milk. Radioactivity was found in the petroleum ether extract of milk at each time interval studied between 4 and 96 hours following a single intravenous dose of 0.02mg/kg or 1mg/kg of ^{14}C-Δ^9-THC given to lactating ewes (Jakubovic et al., 1974). The radioactivity was assumed to be primarily unchanged THC since it has been reported to appear in such an extract (Klausner and Dingell, 1971). This remains to be confirmed. Observations in squirrel monkeys reveal that about 0.2% of a labelled dose of THC appears in the milk during the 24 hours following termination of chronic oral dosing (Chao et al., 1976).

5. Antipsychotics

Perphenazine appears in the milk of lactating ewes within 1 hour after intravenous administration of 0.05 to 1.5mg/kg of the tritiated compound (Shani et al., 1974). As determined by total radioactivity present, levels in the milk of cows and ewes exceeded those in serum within 4 to 6 hours after intramuscular or intravenous injection of the drug. They remained higher in milk for 25 hours after intravenous administration and for 100 hours after intramuscular injection.

Perphenazine is a weakly ionised base (pKa = 7.8) and is both lypophilic and hydrophobic. It thus enters milk in accordance with the pH-pKa passive diffusion concept (Shani et al., 1974). Even though binding to serum was extensive, the drug's high degree of lipid solubility facilitated the rapid passage of the unbound fraction into milk. Because the pH of milk is lower than that of blood, some of the diffusable un-ionised fraction is converted into the ionised form when it enters into milk and perphenazine is consequently 'trapped' in this fluid.

The accumulation of haloperidol is substantially different from that of perphenazine. Concentrations (as determined by radiometric technique) of this compound in milk did not exceed those of serum at any time following intramuscular administration (Ziv et al., 1974). However, concentrations in milk were similar to those in serum 30 hours after injection. Thereafter, the rates of decline in milk and plasma were parallel.

Haloperidol is a water-soluble weak base with a pKa of 8.25 and it has a low (< 20%) protein binding in milk and serum. The predicted M/P ratio for the drug should be 7.2 at equilibrium according to calculations made by Ziv et al. (1974). However, the observed ratio was consistently less than 1.0. It was suggested that this discrepancy occurred because the passage of haloperidol from blood into milk was not via non-ionic passive diffusion. (Our calculation of concentrations achieved by ion partitioning yielded a M/P of 2.1, which is more consistent with experimental findings).

Chlorpromazine, prochlorperazine or trifluoperazine are present in the milk of lactating dogs when these animals are treated chronically with one of these drugs (Flanagan et al., 1959). A peak milk concentration (0.29µg/ml) of chlorpromazine occurred 120 minutes after 1 patient was given a single 1200mg dose (route not specified) of the drug (Blacker et al., 1962). The appearance of this peak in milk lagged behind that observed in plasma (0.75µg/ml at 90 minutes). Chlorpromazine was not detected in milk after a single 600mg dose, but the times at which milk was collected for these measurements was not explicitly stated. (They were probably at 30, 60, 90 and 180 minutes after drug administration.) When a mother was maintained on a schedule of 600mg twice daily for 7 days, chlorpromazine was not detected in the 'morning milk sample' (which morning was not specified).

6. Tricyclic Antidepressants

Although a number of reviews have reported that imipramine does not appear in human breast milk (Knowles, 1965; O'Brien, 1974; Takyi, 1970; White, 1978), one reviewer (Vorherr, 1974b) stated that imipramine is present at a concentration of 1µg/ml milk. However, no citation of the research literature was given for this statement. Apparently, this imipramine concentration in milk was theoretical rather than observed (Vorherr, 1974b). In a misunderstanding of this point, a more recent review (Ananth, 1978) stated that, according to the previous review (Vorherr, 1974b), 'imipramine was excreted in breast milk and that while the drug level in plasma was 0.2 to 1.3mg/100ml, the drug level in milk was 0.1mg'.

Another report further confuses the imipramine-breast milk issue. The International Drug Therapy Newsletter (Ayd, 1973) states that Kahzen et al. (1968) 'published a report on the presence of imipramine metabolites in the milk of nursing rats'. However, only the effect of imipramine on the mammotropic index and body temperature of oestrogen-primed female rats was reported and no data regarding the presence of imipramine metabolites in milk were given.

Also, according to this report (Ayd, 1973), milk supplied by a nursing mother was examined by industrial chemists who found imipramine was present in milk and that its concentrations there were related to the dose given to the mother. Further documentation of this finding is essential.

Other tricyclic antidepressants have been shown to pass into the breast milk of animals and humans. In this regard, excretion of ^{14}C-labelled amitriptyline and nortriptyline into rabbit milk has been reported (Aaes-Jorgensen and Jorgensen, 1977). In this study, the highest concentration of amitriptyline (about 0.5 to 0.7µg/ml) and nortriptyline (0.6 to 0.8µg/ml) in milk occurred at the earlier time intervals studied i.e. at about 1 hour after drug administration (one dose of 2mg/kg for both compounds). The serum concentration for both drugs was above the concentrations in milk until about 6 hours after injection. Beginning at this time and continuing throughout the subsequent times studied (that is, up to 24 hours after drug injection), the M/P ratio for amitriptyline addressed unity, whereas that for nortriptyline was less than unity. These results are at best presumptive since the ratios were based on milk obtained from only 2 rabbits and the variance was large.

Human milk has been examined for amitriptyline (Eschenhof and Rieder, 1969). 5 women received a 50mg oral dose of amitriptyline on the second and third or on the sixth through eighth postpartum days. Milk samples taken immediately before, and 4 and 12 hours after each dose were analysed for amitriptyline and its metabolites. The drug was not found in milk despite an assay sensitivity limit of 0.1µg/ml. Failure to demonstrate amitriptyline in human milk in this study does not exclude its excretion in lactating mothers treated long term for endogenous depression. Steady-state blood concentrations were not obtained since the $t_{1/2\beta}$ for amitriptyline is approximately 32 to 40 hours (Avery, 1976). Also, the daily dose of amitriptyline in some patients is 300mg/day for the treatment of endogenous depression (Byck, 1975).

Dothiepin levels in the milk of 2 lactating mothers were studied (Rees et al., 1976). One 29-year-old woman received 75mg of the drug per day (25mg 3 times daily) for a 3-month period prior to the time that milk samples were drawn. According to these authors, this was adequate time to reach steady-state drug concentrations in plasma. Serum and breast milk samples were collected approximately 3 hours after the second dose of the day. Since dothiepin concentrations were 11µg/ml in the breast milk and 33µg/ml in the maternal serum, the M/P concentration ratio was 0.33.

The second patient received a total of 300mg of dothiepin during a 6-day period and exhibited dothiepin concentrations of 10µg/ml in each fluid. No further details were given with regard to the dosing schedule or the time from last dose to collection of the milk sample.

7. Lithium

Lithium is excreted in human breast milk (Tunnessen and Hertz, 1972; Schou and Amdisen, 1973; Sykes and Quarrie, 1976) and passes freely through the placenta to the fetus (Mackay et al., 1976; Sykes and Quarrie, 1976; Weinstein and Goldfield, 1969). In the 1 case reported by Tunnessen and Hertz (1972), the mother took 600 to 1200mg of lithium carbonate daily. Within a few hours after parturition, the baby became cyanotic, hypotonic, and hypothermic. After warming in an incubator, the cyanosis disappeared and muscle tone improved. Breast feeding was initiated. The infant remained hypotonic during the next 3 days and another episode of hypothermia ensued. Serum lithium concentrations were 1.5mEq/litre in the mother and 0.6mEq/litre in the infant at 5 days of age. Breast milk content was 0.6mEq/litre. Breast feeding was discontinued and lithium concentrations in the infant's serum fell to 0.21mEq/litre by 7 days of age.

On the basis of a literature search as well as some of their own data, Schou and Amdisen (1973) observed that, in 8 cases, lithium concentrations in milk were about half those in the mothers' serum. Other observations included:

(1) During the first week of life the nursing infants' serum lithium levels were approximately half that of the mothers', whereas levels in the milk were about equal to those in the infants' serum; and

(2) During the next 7 weeks of life, the mothers' serum concentration decreased to about 1/3 that of milk and the ratio of levels in milk compared with those in the infants' serum approached 0.20.

An additional report showed that at the time of parturition, when the mother under study was being maintained on a lithium dose of 400mg/day, the lithium concentration in her serum was similar to that in the infant's serum (Sykes and Quarrie, 1976). Serum concentrations in the infant fell progressively during the next 2 weeks despite a marked increase in the concentrations in the mother's serum due to an adjustment of dosage to 600mg/day. At about 18 days after birth, the dose of lithium was increased to 800mg/day and maintained at that level throughout the remainder of the study. Although drug concentrations in breast milk almost doubled from the 14th through to the 28th day following delivery, concentrations in the infant's serum remained essentially constant. At the end of 28 days, the following ratios for lithium concentrations were obtained:

1) Mother's serum/infant's serum, about 6;
2) Maternal M/P = 0.77, and
3) Breast milk/infant's serum, about 2.4.

By 42 days after birth these ratios changed to about 8, 0.25 and 2, respectively. The ratios did not change dramatically from this time to the end of the study at 63 days postpartum.

These data suggest a complex developmentally determined regulation of lithium concentrations in the infant. Also, since the M/P ratio of lithium concentrations in the *one* mother in the study by Sykes and Quarrie (1976) decreased from about 0.77 to 0.25 from day 28 to day 42, the concentrations in milk may be related to factors in addition to the total amount in serum.

8. Antiepileptic Drugs

Phenytoin was found in breast milk of nursing mothers (Horning et al., 1975; Mirkin, 1971; Rane et al., 1974; Svenmark et al., 1960). In a single patient, Svenmark et al. (1960) found a concentration of 6µg/ml in breast milk as compared with 28µg/ml in maternal plasma. The neonatal plasma concentration was not determined. Horning et al. (1975) measured sequential phenytoin concentrations over a 24h period in the milk of a mother who received, for purposes of the study, a single dose of 100mg of phenytoin. The patient ordinarily took 100mg of phenytoin 3 times a day for control of her epilepsy. The initial concentration of phenytoin in a sample obtained 15 minutes before the 100mg dose was 1.7µg/ml. This amount presumably derived from the previous day's medication. Following the 100mg oral dose of phenytoin, the concentration rose to a maximum of 4.2µg/ml at 3 hours and had dropped to 1µg/ml at approximately 6 hours after the dose. The concentration then varied from 0.5 to 1.5µg/ml over the next 18 hours. In this study, neither maternal nor neonatal plasma concentration was measured. The authors suggest that an infant could achieve a therapeutic drug concentration and there is also a chance for enzyme induction in the nursing infant.

Rane et al. (1974) measured phenytoin in maternal and infant plasma and in milk. A plasma level expected from doses delivered via milk was calculated. Four nursing infants showed a low plateau of phenytoin in plasma. Nadir levels in milk and maternal plasma, 12 hours after 250mg phenytoin per day, were 0.26 and 0.58µg/ml respectively. The M/P ratio was 0.45. Peak milk level (3h post dose) was 0.58µg/ml. An average milk level of 4µg/ml was estimated for another mother. Based on daily dose of phenytoin and a Vd for adults, her infant's plasma level was calculated to be 0.4µg/ml as compared with an observed 0.5µg/ml after six days of dosing.

In an earlier study, Livingston (1956) reported that none of the nursing infants of 28 epileptic women taking either 300 or 600mg per day of phenytoin became drowsy or lethargic, but 1 child in another study developed methaemoglobinaemia while his mother was taking phenobarbitone and phenytoin for epilepsy (Illingworth, 1953). The child's symptoms disappeared when breast feeding was discontinued.

Milk and plasma levels of carbamazepine and carbamazepine epoxide were measured in three women (Pynonnen, 1975 and 1977). The M/P ratio was 0.6 for the parent drug and 1.05 for its epoxide metabolite. The metabolite was detected 3 days after birth in the infants' plasma and at 3 to 5 weeks, in two of the three infants. Plasma levels of carbamazepine in the children were 30 to 50% of maternal plasma. No adverse effects were noted in the nursing infants.

The M/P ratio for multiple antiepileptic drugs has recently been described by Kaneko et al. (1979). This ratio was determined from mean plasma levels obtained 3 to 32 days post partum in those women being treated with antiepileptic drugs chronically. The mean (± S.D.) M/P ratios were: phenytoin, 0.18 ± 0.06, phenobarbital 0.46 ± 0.25, primidone 0.81 ± 0.18, carbamazepine 0.39 ± 0.19, ethosuximide 0.79 ± 0.33. The marked interindividual variation was emphasized, but the ratios generally agree with those previously reported. Notable deviations include a lower ratio for carbamazepine, 0.39 compared to 0.60 (Pynnonen et al., 1975, 1977). Marked variation in the ratio for phenobarbital was ascribed to its PK_a 7.2 and the effect of changes in milk pH. An infant dose of 16.5mg of phenobarbital per day was estimated for one woman who had a plasma level of 33µg/ml. These workers advocate correlative studies for breast milk and saliva as one means of deriving milk levels where maternal plasma levels are known. [See also review by Rane (1978)].

7

Alcohol

Helmut M. Redetzki

Many babies are intermittently, periodically or chronically exposed to alcohol through breast feeding. Consumption of alcoholic beverages has become universally and socially acceptable except for views held by a few opposing cultural and religious groups. Unfortunately, permissive attitudes have contributed to a high prevalence of compulsive drinking and alcoholism. These attitudes and a lack of information about the acute or prolonged effects of alcohol in the neonate weaken attempts to limit alcohol consumption in the breast feeding woman.

While most available data describe only ethanol, it must be understood that alcoholic beverages are rarely pure but contain various congeners and byproducts of fermentation (e.g. fusel oils). These, as well as some of the metabolic products of ethanol, are probably transferred into milk. The significance of these substances in infant morbidity is unknown and remains unassessed.

Ethanol passes readily through cell membranes and distributes freely in the body water space. This explains its occurrence in milk. Comparing the average water content of human milk with that of blood (approximately 88% versus 85%), one would expect that the alcohol concentration of human milk should equal or slightly exceed that of blood. Not all data confirm this assumption, especially if hind rather than fore milk samples are used. Many of the older studies (before 1930) are unreliable as alcohol determinations in the 'pre-Widmark' era suffered from methodological difficulties and lack of specificity (Gruner, 1967). The latter objection was mainly overcome in the early 1950's with the introduction of the enzymatic analysis of

Table VIII. Ethanol and acetaldehyde content of milk and peripheral blood of lactating women

Sample[1]	Time			
	30m	60m	90m	120m
	Ethanol (μmol/ml)			
Blood	19.1 ± 6.5[2]	18.2 ± 2.5	15.0 ± 2.1	12.4 ± 2.4
Milk	15.8 ± 5.4	16.9 ± 2.5	14.1 ± 2.5	11.3 ± 2.6
	Acetaldehyde[3] (μmol/ml)			
Blood	44.4 ± 21.1	31.5 ± 13.7	26.7 ± 10.5	19.3 ± 7.5

1 Samples were obtained at the stated time intervals after peroral administration of 0.6g of ethanol per kg maternal body weight.
2 All results are given as means ± standard deviation of 12 experiments.
3 Acetaldehyde was not detected in milk.

ethanol (Bucher and Redetzki, 1951) and in the 1960's with the development of reliable gas chromatographic methods (Maricq and Molle, 1959). Only the more recent studies will be reviewed in detail. Most older studies cited by Sollmann (1957) and Kesaniemi (1974) are of anecdotal value only.

The most valuable study is that of Kesaniemi (1974) who measured ethanol and acetaldehyde in the milk and peripheral blood of lactating women at predetermined intervals after the peroral administration of 0.6g of ethanol/kg of body weight. The subjects received the alcohol in the morning after an overnight fasting period. It was provided as a 15% (w/v) solution in water and consumed within 5 minutes. Blood samples were taken from the antecubital vein 30, 60, 90, and 120 minutes after ethanol administration. Milk samples were obtained by milking the breasts at the same times. The samples were analysed by gas chromatography using the head space technique. Table VIII summarises the data. Ethanol absorption was very rapid under the conditions of this study. Maximum blood concentrations occurred between 30 and 60 minutes. Alcohol concentrations in the milk were similar to those in plasma although the data suggest a lag phase for the distribution of alcohol into milk. During the terminal decay phase comparable concentrations in the blood and milk were maintained. However, at all the times studied, the average concentration of alcohol in milk was below that in blood with a milk to plasma ratio of 0.9. This finding could relate to the fat content of milk and concurrent changes in milk water as well as to the rate of distribution to and from the milk compartment. The observation that acetaldehyde, the major metabolite of ethanol, is not excreted in milk is significant since some have postulated that acetaldehyde contributes to the toxicity of alcohol.

That alcohol taken in moderation by a nursing mother does not discernibly or adversely affect her infant is a viewpoint expressed by many investigators. Since reliable data on blood alcohol concentrations of breast-fed infants are lacking, it is helpful to assess the problem on a projected intake basis. Assuming that a 4-month-old infant who weighs 6.8kg drinks 180ml of milk in 1 nursing and that his body water is 0.65 litre/kg of body weight, one can (using the milk/maternal blood alcohol ratio of 0.9) not only assess the average amount of alcohol ingested, but also get an approximation of the maximum blood alcohol concentration which results from a single feeding. Calculating these data for 3 representative levels of maternal alcohol exposure and concomitant nursing, one derives the following conclusions:

1) Blood alcohol concentration of 50mg/dl (moderate social drinking: i.e. 2 to 3 cocktails, 2 to 3 glasses of wine or 2 to 3 340ml bottles of beer). Amount of alcohol received by the infant is 82mg (12mg/kg); maximum blood alcohol concentration of the infant is insignificant (1.9mg/dl).

2) Blood alcohol concentration of 100mg/dl (heavier, probably habitual drinking). Amount of alcohol received by the infant is 164mg (24mg/kg); maximum blood alcohol concentration of the infant is insignificant (3.7mg/dl).

3) Blood alcohol concentration of 300mg/dl (probably the highest blood alcohol concentration at which a mother could nurse her child). Amount of alcohol received by infant is 492mg (72mg/kg); maximum alcohol concentration of infant is 11.1mg/dl. This could cause mild sedation.

Beyond these more commonly applicable values, a few early and unusual observations have been recorded in the literature. One describes the highest milk alcohol level: 560mg/dl (Frontali, 1915). The other is a report (Bisdom, 1937) which describes symptoms of alcohol intoxication in an 8-day-old breast-fed infant whose mother consumed a whole bottle of port wine. The child was in deep sleep from which it could not be readily awakened. Infant respirations were slow and snoring, pupils reacted only slightly to light, and the pulse was rapid and weak.

Two additional reports describe adverse effects in breast-fed infants nursed by mothers who drank chronically and excessively. The description by Hoh (1969) of severe hypoprothrombinaemic bleeding in breast-fed young infants is based on a study of 23 full-term Chinese infants whose ages ranged from 21 to 60 days. They were admitted during a period of 5 years to the Singapore General Hospital. All had abnormally long clotting times (8 to over 20 minutes) and prothrombin times of 24 to 90 seconds, but normal platelet counts. Plasma fibrinogen, determined in 2 infants was normal. All were breast-fed by mothers who had been drinking alcohol in the form of tonic wine, rice wine, or brandy, in amounts varying between 12 and 16 'drachmas of alcohol' daily. Alcohol, ingested with the mothers' milk, presumably contributed to the infants' bleeding by depressing their hepatic prothrombin synthesis.

In the second report, Binkiewicz et al. (1978) described the development of a pseudo-Cushing syndrome in a 4-month-old female infant breast-fed by a mother who consumed excessive amounts of alcohol. A random check of her milk revealed an alcohol concentration of 100mg/dl. From approximately 8 weeks of age the infant gained weight at an increased rate. At the age of 4 months she was markedly obese and had a strikingly moon shaped facial appearance, but virilisation was not noted. Laboratory tests confirmed the diagnosis and revealed increased excretion of free cortisol in the urine and impaired suppression of cortisol secretion by dexamethasone. While this syndrome is well recognised in adult alcoholics (Smals et al., 1976), this is the first report of its occurrence in an infant. The relationship to maternal alcohol ingestion is convincing since the symptoms disappeared rapidly after the mother discontinued ethanol ingestion.

In addition to possible direct, harmful effects on the infant, some consideration must be given to experimental data which indicate that ingestion of relatively large amounts of alcohol (1 to 2g/kg) leads to a significant reduction o the milk ejection reflex in lactating mothers (Cobo, 1973). The mechanism of the depression can be explained by an alcohol-induced inhibition of oxytocin release (Wagner and Fuchs, 1968).

In summary, one can conclude that ethanol is freely secreted into milk in concentrations slightly below those in blood. Milk alcohol concentrations decrease in parallel with those in blood during the elimination phase but appear to lag during the absorption phase. There is no evidence that occasional moderate ingestion of alcohol by the mother is harmful to the infant. Intoxicated mothers should not breast feed their babies and chronic alcoholic mothers who will not stop drinking should be discouraged from breast feeding.

8

Antimicrobials

R. Don Brown

Little is known about risks to nursing infants incurred by antibiotic consumption via breast milk. For example, chloramphenicol is contraindicated in the nursing mother (Abramowicz, 1979), presumably because it produces milk concentrations equivalent to '50% of the maternal serum levels and high enough to cause bone marrow depression in the infants' (Hervada et al., 1978). This opinion is based on studies of a very limited number of nursing mothers.

There is also a paucity of information of a kinetic nature concerning the passage of other antibiotics into human breast milk. Limited studies have determined concentrations of an antibiotic simultaneously in plasma and milk. However, these studies yield only one or a few experimental M/P concentration ratios under variable conditions of milk sampling. It is not possible to derive a general or drug specific kinetic model from such studies.

Theoretical information about antibiotic concentrations in breast milk can be derived from the concept of pH partition and ion trapping (table IX). Although this information is of general value, it does not give an accurate representation of drug concentrations in whole milk. The percentage of the drug which is bound to plasma proteins and to milk proteins, the binding affinity or capacity, and the possibility of active transport are not considered. Milk composition and variable pH of the milk (both dependent on the breast feeding pattern) also affect the amount of drug excreted. Additionally, metabolites may have a role in the production of toxicity and they could have different characteristics (pK and lipid partition coefficients) which affect their excretion in milk as compared with the parent drug.

The penicillins and cephalosporins are apparently excreted in milk in relatively low concentrations, the M/P ratios being in the order of 0 to 0.2 for drugs in these classes (Greene et al., 1946; Knowles, 1965; Lipman, 1977; Voshioka et al., 1979). These ratios are much lower than would be expected based solely on pH partitioning and ion trapping (table IX) and indicate that other factors, such as plasma versus milk protein binding or active transport, have played a major role in the distribution of these drugs into milk. Rasmussen (1959), using cows and goats, found that, after correcting for protein binding, the experimental ultrafiltrate ratio of benzylpenicillin

Table IX. Theoretical M/P ultrafiltrate ratios of selected antibiotics

Drug	Nature[1]	pKa[2]	Predicted M/P[3]	
			milk pH 7.0	milk pH 7.25
Penicillins				
Ampicillin	A	2.5	0.45	0.79
	A	7.2	0.68	0.88
Penicillin G	A	2.7	0.45	0.79
Methicillin	A	3	0.45	0.79
Oxacillin	A	2.9	0.45	0.79
Carbenicillin	A	3.3	0.45	0.79
Cephalosporins				
Cephalothin	A	2.5	0.45	0.79
Cephalexin	A	2.5	0.45	0.79
	A	7.3	0.71	0.89
Cephaloridine	A	4.75	0.45	0.79
Tetracyclines				
Tetracycline	B	3.3	1	1
	B	7.7	1.86	1.18
	B	9.7	2.23	1.26
Chlortetracycline	B	2.85	1	1
Rolitetracycline	B	7.4	1.65	1.14
Lincomycin	B	7.6	1.79	1.17
Clindamycin	B	7.45	1.69	1.14
Erythromycin	B	8.8	2.2	1.25
Aminoglycosides				
Gentamicin	B	8.2	2.09	1.23
Kanamycin	B	7.2	1.51	1.11
Sulphonamides				
Sulphadiazine	A	6.4	0.5	0.82
Sulphamethoxazole	A	5.7	0.46	0.8
Sulphadimidine	A	7.4	0.74	0.9
Sulphadimethoxine	A	5.9	0.47	0.8
Trimethoprim	B	6.4	1.12	1.03

1 A = acid; B = base.
2 All pKa values were obtained from Avery (1976a).
3 Plasma pH = 7.35.

(0.25) agreed with the ratio calculated on the basis of pH partition and ion trapping (0.16). This value is different from that for the human because of species differences in plasma and milk pH.

The theoretical M/P ratio calculated for tetracycline is somewhat similar to that found in human studies. The theoretical values range from 1 to 2.23 (table IX) and the observed values reported are 0.6 to 0.8 (Vorherr, 1974b). At a dosage of 500mg orally every six hours for 3 days the milk to plasma ratio ranged between 0.6 and 0.8, but tetracycline was not detectable in infant plasma — the detection limit of the assay being 0.05µg/ml. The relative achlorhydria of newborns may possibly decrease solubility of tetracycline and hence its absorption (Posner, 1954, 1955). Accordingly, adverse effects have not been reported in the nursing infant from administration of any of the tetracyclines to their mothers. However, it is theoretically possible that staining of teeth or delayed bone growth could occur. As a consequence, Hervada et al. (1978) recommends that the 'potential for this side effect should be considered and alternate therapy prescribed if possible'.

Lincomycin has an observed M/P ratio of about 0.15 (Vorherr, 1974b) compared with its theoretical ratio of 1.2 to 1.8 (table IX) which agrees with that (1.9-4.3) found for cows (Rasmussen, 1966a; Gyrd-Hansen and Rasmussen, 1967). The reason for this discrepancy is not known. White (1978) stated that the concentrations of both lincomycin and clindamycin in breast milk were insignificant and there was no effect on the infant. The same type of assertion is made for erythromycin (White, 1978) which has an observed M/P ratio of 0.5 (Knowles, 1965) or 2.5 to 3.0 (Vorherr, 1974b). The calculated ultrafiltrate M/P ratio for erythromycin is 2.2 for a milk pH of 7.0.

The aminoglycoside antibiotics are generally considered safe drugs to use in nursing mothers. However, the observed M/P ratios for kanamycin and streptomycin range from 0.4 to 1.0 (Vorherr, 1974b). Aminoglycosides are very poorly absorbed from the gastrointestinal tract and this minimises the chance of adverse effects (e.g. ototoxicity, nephrotoxicity) from drug delivered via breast milk. Gastrointestinal tract inflammation or diarrhoea in the infant may increase absorption. Serum concentrations of aminoglycoside antibiotics in such nursing infants have not been measured to substantiate this concern.

The sulphonamide antibacterials have observed M/P ratios of 0.2 to 0.97 for cows and goats (Rasmussen, 1958). These values are in agreement with the theoretical ratios (table IX) and an observed ratio of 1.0 for sulphapyridine in man (Vorherr, 1974b). As a consequence, the risk for hyperbilirubinaemic encephalopathy is enhanced, as is the risk for haemolytic anaemia in infants with glucose-6-phosphate dehydrogenase deficiency. One case of haemolytic anaemia has been reported (White, 1978).

Chloramphenicol has an observed M/P ratio of about 0.50 (Smadel el al., 1949). At least 50 % of the drug in milk is present as an inactive metabolite without antibacterial activity (Havelka et al., 1968). As previously stated, the use of this drug in nursing mothers is contraindicated.

9

Bronchodilators and Antiallergy Drugs

Bettina C. Hilman

With the possible exception of theophylline (Yurchak and Jusko, 1976), a review of the literature on the excretion of drugs in breast milk (Catz and Giacola, 1972; Hervada, 1978; Knowles, 1965, 1972, 1973, 1974; Vorherr, 1974b; White, 1978) reveals little information on the pharmacokinetics of bronchodilators or other drugs used in the management of allergy. Nevertheless, the use of such drugs is often necessary, even if the patient is nursing her infant. The extent to which bronchodilators and other antiallergic drugs are excreted in breast milk needs to be better defined, since this information would answer the critical question: Is the drug-related risk to the infant sufficient to warrant discontinuation of nursing?

1. Antihistamines and Antihistamine-Decongestants

Although quantitative determinations of antihistaminic drugs in breast milk have not been reported, qualitative tests have documented the excretion of diphenhydramine, trimeprazine, and tripelennamine in human milk. However, no severe adverse effects have been reported in the nursing infant (O'Brien, 1974).

Mortimer (1977) has recently reported symptoms of irritability, excessive crying and disturbed sleep patterns of 5 days duration in a breast-fed infant whose mother had been given a long acting oral antihistamine decongestant for allergic rhinitis. The mother began taking this medication (6mg of dexbrompheniramine maleate and

120mg of d-isoephedrine sulphate per dose) twice daily about 2 days before the onset of symptoms in her breast fed infant. The dosing schedule was continued throughout the infant's 5 symptomatic days. Resumption of normal behaviour by the infant occurred within 12 hours after this medication was discontinued by the mother and an artificial formula was given for 2 feedings.

2. Corticosteroids

Although corticosteroid excretion in breast milk and its effects on the nursing infant have not been adequately studied in man, some animal studies have been reported. Severe adverse effects on postnatal development of suckling rats were seen after maternal administration of 20mg cortisone per day during pregnancy or lactation (Mercier-Parot, 1955). Katz and Duncan (1975a,b) reported concentrations of 0.16 and 2.67µg/dl of prednisolone and prednisone, respectively, in breast milk 2 hours after 10mg of prednisone was given to a nursing woman for the treatment of iridocyclitis. 7 healthy lactating volunteers were given 5mg of radioisotope-labelled prednisolone (McKenzie et al., 1975). Milk samples were obtained for 48 hours after dosing. An initial rapid and then asymptotic decay profile was found for radioactivity in milk. An average of 0.14% of the dose was recovered in a litre of milk. A very small prednisone dose would thus be delivered via milk to the infant.

The long term effects of corticosteroids have not been documented and appropriate studies have not been carried out on the pharmacokinetics of these compounds in breast milk. Some authors (Knowles, 1974) consider breast feeding as contraindicated in women given these drugs, but rat studies form the basis for this opinion.

3. Adrenaline (epinephrine)

Since adrenaline (epinephrine) is destroyed during its passage through the gastrointestinal tract, its appearance in breast milk is considered unlikely (Catz and Giacoia, 1972).

4. β-Adrenoceptor Agonist Bronchodilators

The human milk content of isoprenaline (isoproterenol), isoetharine, or the newer β_2-adrenoceptor agonists such as orciprenaline (metaproterenol), terbutaline, salbutamol (albuterol) and fenoterol has not been described. At the present time there are no readily available methods of monitoring serum concentrations of β_2-adrenoceptor agonist bronchodilators. Since no quantitative studies of these agents in nursing mothers have been reported, the distribution of these drugs into breast milk

Table X. Some pharmacological properties of β-adrenoceptor agonist bronchodilators

Drug	Molecular weight	pKa	Plasma half-life (h)	Protein binding (%)	Route of administration[1]	Relative duration of action[2]
Isoprenaline (isoproterenol)	211.24	8.6, 10.1, 12.0	2.5		I (PA; NS); IV; O	+
Isoetharine	239.31				I (PA; NS); O	+ +
Orciprenaline (metaproterenol)	211.27	8.8; 11.8	1.5	10	I (PA; NS); IV; O	+ + +
Terbutaline	225.29	10.1	3-4	25	I (PA); SC; O	+ + + +
Salbutamol (albuterol)	239.31	9.3; 10.3	2-4		O; I (PA; NS); IV	+ + + +
Fenoterol	303.37				I (PA)	+ + + +

1 I = inhalation; PA = pressurised aerosol; NS = nebulised solution; O = orally; IV = intravenously; SC = subcutaneously.
2 Duration of action relative to that of isoprenaline (2.5h).

can only be postulated from what is known about the pharmacology and chemical characteristics of each drug (table X).

Isoprenaline (isoproterenol) is the prototype of the β-adrenoceptor stimulants. It is a potent bronchodilator when administered by aerosol, and it is rapidly metabolised by catechol-O-methyltransferase (COMT) after inhalation (van As, 1975). After oral administration, it is converted by gastrointestinal sulphatases to an ethereal sulphate, thus rendering it inactive by this route (van As, 1975). Because of its very short half-life (2.5 hours), it should not have prolonged concentrations in maternal plasma after the usual therapeutic doses. Excretion of significant quantities into breast milk is not expected.

The newer β-adrenoceptor agonists were developed to increase the duration of bronchodilator activity and to minimise cardiac activity (i.e. more β₂-selective). The particle size of the aerosol in addition to the dose determine the concentration of these drugs in maternal plasma. The larger the aerosol particles, the more likely they are to be deposited in the upper airways (trachea and pharynx) and thus facilitate absorption into the blood stream (van As, 1975). The smaller particle size aerosols tend to be distributed more evenly into the mother's smaller airways where they are able to achieve bronchodilation at a lower dosage (van As, 1975). Theoretically, administration of the newer β-adrenoceptor stimulants by smaller particle size aerosol should reduce the amount of these drugs which appear in breast milk.

Isoetharine, one of the first of the β-adrenergic stimulants developed to improve β₂-selectivity, is used mainly by inhalation and has a similar time of onset but longer duration of action than isoprenaline. Its metabolic fate is similar to that of isoprenaline.

Orciprenaline (metaproterenol), a resorcinol derivative of isoprenaline, has 2 hydroxyl groups attached at the meta (3, 5) positions on the phenyl ring rather than 1 at the meta position and 1 at the para (4) position. This structural difference accounts for its resistance to COMT or sulphatases, thus explaining its longer duration of action. It is effective by oral administration for about 4 hours and by inhalation for 2 to 5 times longer than isoproterenol (Avner, 1975; Jack, 1978; van As, 1975). Thus it would persist in maternal plasma longer and be more readily available for excretion into breast milk. The peak bronchodilator action after oral administration occurs 1 to 2 hours after administration (Avner, 1975; Jack, 1978; van As, 1975). The peak absorption into maternal plasma is also presumed to occur during this period. Little has been published about the metabolism of this drug.

Orciprenaline is the parent compound of terbutaline, an N-tertiary butyl homologue (van As, 1975), and also of fenoterol. Terbutaline is an effective bronchodilator when given by inhalation, orally, or by subcutaneous injection. It has more β_2-selectivity than orciprenaline (Avner, 1975; Jack et al., 1978; van As, 1975). It is also resistant to COMT and sulphatase. Bronchodilation begins within 5 minutes after inhalation and is maintained as long as 5 hours. Administration of terbutaline by subcutaneous injection causes bronchodilation which is maintained for 2 to 3 hours or longer. Oral terbutaline has an onset of action within 30 minutes and persists for at least 5 hours; only about 50% is reported to be absorbed. Most of the absorbed drug is converted into a sulphate ester, which is excreted together with the unchanged drug in the urine (Jack et al., 1978).

Fenoterol, a p-hydroxyphenyl derivative, is a more potent and selective bronchodilator than its parent compound, orciprenaline (Avner, 1975; Jack et al., 1978; van As, 1975). It has a similar bronchodilator action to that of terbutaline.

Salbutamol (albuterol), a saligenin derivative of isoprenaline with an N-tertiary substituent on the side chain, is an effective bronchodilator. It has a peak action about 15 minutes after inhalation and this persists for 4 to 6 hours (Avner, 1975; Jack et al., 1978; van As, 1975). After inhalation, it is slowly absorbed and only small amounts are found in the plasma (Avner, 1975). It is well absorbed from the intestinal tract and rapidly excreted in the urine (Avner, 1975).

5. Theophylline and Related Compounds

Recently, Yurchak and Jusko (1976) reported adverse reactions in an infant receiving theophylline in breast milk. They also reported results of studies on the pharmacokinetics of theophylline in plasma and breast milk. A 24-year-old nursing mother received aminophylline tablets every 6 hours for control of her asthma. Her breast-fed infant showed irritability, fretfulness, and insomnia only on the days when the mother was receiving aminophylline. These adverse effects in the infant occurred repeatedly over 9 months. During this period, samples of breast milk contained significant concentrations of theophylline. Pharmacokinetic studies on this woman and 4 other subjects revealed that theophylline distributes well into breast milk with the average M/P drug concentration ratio of 0.7. An approximate 2 hour lag for the time to maximum concentration was seen for milk compared with serum (fig. 18). A mono-exponential decay was not apparent for theophylline in milk, although both the serum and milk concentrations decreased rapidly from 3 to 6 hours after drug administration (see also section 4.12). Based on relative body weights, these authors postulate that the infant of a nursing mother would usually receive less than 10% of the mother's dose of theophylline.

Theophylline pharmacokinetics were studied in 5 nursing women: 3 received a single dose of 4.25mg/kg of theophylline as aminophylline in solution, and 2 others received multiple doses of 200mg of aminophylline 4 times daily (Yurchak and Jusko, 1976). The 2 patients receiving multiple doses also received 15 to 20mg of prednisone on the day of the study. Theophylline concentrations in blood, milk and saliva samples were measured by a high pressure liquid chromatography technique (Jusko and Poliszezuk, 1975; Thompson et al., 1974) which is specific for theophylline. Protein binding determinations were carried out by ultrafiltration techniques using serum and milk. The percentage of protein binding of theophylline in serum in these 5 nursing women ranged from 42 to 69%, while the percentage of

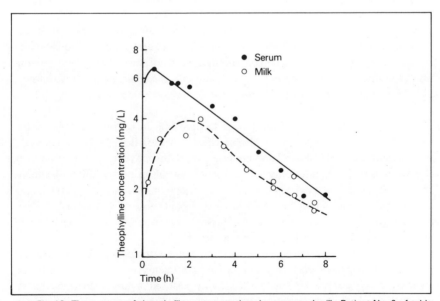

Fig. 18. Time course of theophylline concentrations in serum and milk. Patient No. 2 of table XI received 4.25mg/kg aminophylline in solution orally (revised from Yurchak and Jusko, 1976).

Table XI. Milk to serum concentration ratios of theophylline[1]

Patient	Dosage[2]	Milk: serum[3]	Milk pH	% Protein bound	
				serum	milk
1	SD	0.73	7.60	50	0
2	SD	0.61	7.65	55	1
3	SD	—	—	—	—
4	MD	0.87	6.70	42	0
5	MD	0.63	6.35	69	24

1 Modified from data of Yurchak and Jusko (1976).
2 SD = single dose; MD = multiple dose.
3 Calculated from the ratio of the respective areas under the serum concentration-time curve (AUC).

protein-bound theophylline in milk ranged from 0 to 24 %. The pH of the breast milk in these 5 women ranged from 6.35 to 7.65 with an average of 7.08.

The plasma half-life of theophylline in nursing mothers in the studies of Yurchak and Jusko (1976) varied from 3.7 to 8 hours with a mean of 5.6 hours. The time to peak milk concentration ranged from 1 to 3 hours. The apparent volume of distribution in 2 of these nursing women receiving a single dose of theophylline was found to be 0.49 and 0.45L/kg. A plasma half-life of 4 and 8 hours was found in the 2 patients, respectively. The M/P concentration ratios of theophylline for 5 nursing women in this study are listed in table XI. 4 nursing asthmatic mothers (patient nos. 2 and 5 in table XI) treated with theophylline, did not observe any irritability in their children.

Analysis of the pharmacokinetics of theophylline in serum and milk of the mother whose infant experienced adverse effects revealed that she had a relatively short plasma half-life (4 hours) and her peak serum theophylline concentration was attained within 30 minutes after the administration of an oral solution of amino-phylline (fig. 18). The peak concentration of theophylline was 6.8mg/litre in the maternal serum and 4.0mg/litre in milk after a single dose of 4.25mg/kg of theophylline. Apparently, consumption of milk with this concentration of theophylline was enough to produce mild symptoms in her infant.

Theophylline products which have more rapid rates of absorption reach an earlier and higher peak plasma concentration than theophylline preparations which are more slowly absorbed (Koup, 1978). Highly perfused organs, such as the breast, are exposed to higher concentrations when the theophylline concentration is higher in the plasma. Less rapidly absorbed theophylline preparations may be advisable for nursing mothers in order to avoid the higher peak concentrations in maternal plasma and the resultant higher concentrations in breast milk.

The relationship between theophylline dosing interval and frequency of breast feeding has not been studied with regard to drug concentration in milk. Back diffusion of drug from the mammary gland would reduce the amount of drug in the milk when the interval between drug ingestion and breast feeding is increased and maternal plasma drug concentration declines. A high concentration or prolonged presence of the drug in the maternal circulation would tend to enhance its passage into breast milk. Sustained release theophylline preparations for the control of asthma and other forms of chronic obstructive airways disease are being used more widely. This could place nursing infants at increased risk for high amounts consumed and for consequent adverse effects of this drug.

Higher doses of theophylline than those recommended in the past, are currently being prescribed as it has been found that optimum bronchodilation is achieved with serum concentrations between 10 and 20mg/litre. About 8mg (or 2mg/kg/day for a 4kg infant) is the estimated maximum amount of theophylline which an infant could ingest by consuming 1 litre of breast milk per day. This assumes that the mother achieved a peak serum concentration of about 12mg/litre on a daily dosage regimen of 16mg/kg/day of theophylline and nursed her infant near the time of peak concentrations (Yurchak and Jusko, 1976). Small infants who metabolise the drug slowly may accumulate a significant plasma concentration of theophylline in relation to body weight. Aranda et al. (1976) reported a mean plasma half-life of theophylline in premature infants 3 to 15 days of age of 30.2 $\pm$ 6.5h with a range of 14.4 to 57.7h. Kadlec et al. (1978) reported a mean half-life of 4.92 $\pm$ 1.88h in a group of children whose ages ranged from 3 months to 6 years.

Nursing mothers who require theophylline for control of symptoms of airways obstruction should also avoid ingestion of theobromine from chocolate. Resman et al. (1977) have studied the pharmacokinetics of theobromine, another member of the methylxanthine group of drugs, in a group of 6 nursing mothers. They found the pharmacokinetics of this drug similar to those of theophylline. Theobromine is present in chocolate and in all cocoa products. This study confirmed that theobromine passes freely into human milk following the ingestion of chocolate. Theobromine is eliminated with a mean plasma half-life of 7.1h compared with 5.6h for theophylline. The body clearance of theobromine ranged from 37 to 89ml/kg/h (x $\pm$ SD = 65 $\pm$ 20ml/kg/h) and the apparent volume of distribution varied from 0.44 to 0.82L/kg (x $\pm$ SD = 0.62 $\pm$ 0.13L/kg). Theobromine is only 15 to 25% bound to plasma protein, whereas protein binding of theophylline in plasma ranged from 42 to 69%. The protein binding of theobromine in milk was 0 to 24% with a mean M/P ratio of 0.82 (range of 0.60 to 1.06). Theobromine in chocolate had an average absorption half-life ($t_{1/2abs}$) of 0.5 $\pm$ 0.1h. The maximum theobromine concentration in plasma was attained between 1.5 and 3.1h after ingestion of chocolate, whereas the maximum concentration in milk was reached after 2.1 to 3.3h. Similar concentrations and an apparent parallel decay pattern were noted for theobromine in milk and plasma from 4 to 14 hours after dosing. Drug concentrations in milk obtained concomitantly from the right and left breast were similar.

Based on the average data from this study (Resman et al., 1977), the infant of a nursing mother who ingested 4oz of chocolate (240mg of theobromine) every 6 hours would be exposed to about 10mg theobromine per day or 1 to 2mg/kg/day. This might be sufficient to produce clinical effects in some sensitive individuals. With the slower metabolism of theophylline and related drugs in premature and very young infants, cumulative effects of both theobromine and theophylline may be responsible for adverse effects in some infants of nursing mothers.

The pharmacokinetic information on theobromine and theophylline in breast milk is important to the physician treating the asthmatic patient who requires theophylline preparations for control of her asthma and who also wishes to nurse her infant. Although either drug alone would not appear in breast milk in pharmacologically significant amounts for most infants, the additive effect of both could conceivably produce adverse effects. Assessment of additive effects should also include caffeine consumed in coffee, colas, tea, and other foods (see section 6.1.3).

10

Anticoagulant and Cardiovascular Drugs

John W. Dailey

There is a lack of detailed scientific studies concerned with the rate and amount of anticoagulant or cardiovascular drug passage into breast milk. Most information about drug excretion into human breast milk is from case reports on very limited patient populations. Very few systematic studies have been performed to relate drug concentration in the mother's blood and milk to blood concentrations and therapeutic or toxic effects in the infant. Based on the concept of pH partition and ion trapping, several drugs in these 2 classes might be expected to be at least as concentrated in an ultrafiltrate of breast milk as in an ultrafiltrate of plasma (table XII).

1. Anticoagulants

Warfarin was measured in the plasma and breast milk of 13 mothers by methods sensitive enough to detect $0.08\mu mol$ per litre ($25ng/ml$) [Orme et al., 1977]. Warfarin was not found in breast milk even though the plasma warfarin concentration averaged $4.0\mu mol/litre$ (range 1.6 to $8.5\mu mol/litre$). 7 of the 13 mothers were breast feeding their infants, none of whom showed detectable plasma concentrations of warfarin. Also, in 4 of the 7 infants, clotting time was within normal limits or less than the mother's clotting time. Warfarin was judged safe for use by nursing mothers, but it was emphasised that the data applied only to warfarin and not to other anticoagulants. Based on its physicochemical characteristics, this finding for warfarin

Table XII. Predicted ultrafiltrate M/P ratio for selected anticoagulant and cardiovascular drugs

Drug	pKa[1]	Predicted M/P ratios[2]	
		milk pH 7.0	milk pH 7.25
Basic drugs			
Hydrallazine	7.1	1.45	1.10
Lignocaine (lidocaine)	7.9	1.96	1.20
Clonidine	8.25	2.10	1.23
Phenytoin	8.3	2.11	1.23
Procainamide	9.2	2.22	1.26
Propranolol	9.45	2.23	1.26
Acidic Drugs			
Dicoumarol	5.7	0.46	0.80
Warfarin	5.05	0.45	0.80
Frusemide (furosemide)	3.8	0.79	0.45

1   pKa was obtained from Avery (1976a).
2   A plasma pH 7.35 was used.

is not unexpected. Warfarin is a weakly acidic drug (pKa 5.05) and is highly bound (approximately 97%) to plasma proteins. Because it is a weak acid it will be highly ionised (> 99%) in plasma at pH 7.35. It would also be extensively ionised in milk but to a lesser extent than in plasma. With so little of the drug non-protein-bound and with even less in the nonionised form, it is not surprising that little warfarin crosses the lipid barrier from plasma into milk. A similar argument can be supported for dicoumarol, which is also a weak acid (pKa 5.7) and is highly bound (95%) to plasma proteins. Dicoumarol was administered to 125 nursing mothers without altering pro-thrombin activity in the infants (Bambel and Hunter, 1950). Drug concentrations in breast milk and in mother's and infant's blood were not measured in this early study. Absence of clotting time alterations in mother and infant suggested that therapeutic concentrations were not achieved in the nursing infants.

Heparin is also reported to be safe to use in nursing mothers. It is too large a molecule (MW 17,000) to cross lipid barriers and is thus not excreted in breast milk (Hervada et al., 1978; see section 4.5).

Insufficient documentation exists for effects on the infant from other antico-agulants when used during nursing. A phenindione-treated mother nursed an infant who developed a haematoma following surgery for repair of a scrotal hernia. The infant's prothrombin time was 50% of normal but returned to normal following the necessary therapeutic interventions and cessation of breast feeding (Eckstein and Jack, 1970). This is the only case reported for this drug. Since more extensive studies have indicated that warfarin and dicoumarol are safe for use during nursing, this 1 case may be enough to suggest that phenindione not be used during nursing and alternative drugs be selected.

The drug which has caused the most confusion among anticoagulants given to breast feeding mothers is ethylbiscoumacetate (Hervada et al, 1978). Illingworth and Finch (1959) found no adverse effects in 22 healthy breast-fed mothers who were receiving this drug. Additionally, in 38 specimens of maternal milk that they examined only 13 were found to have detectable concentrations of ethylbiscoumacetate and the highest concentration found was only 6% of the average maternal plasma concentrations. Other authors have found what appeared to be an unidentified active metabolite of ethylbiscoumacetate in the milk of nursing mothers who were taking the drug (Gostof et al, 1952). This unidentified metabolite may have led to the unusually high rate of bleeding problems (5 of 42 infants) in this study. At any rate, the controversy surrounding this drug still exists and, since there are safe alternative drugs, its use in nursing mothers should probably be avoided.

2. Cardiac Glycosides

Measurements of digoxin concentrations in maternal and infant plasma and in breast milk have been performed recently (Chan et al., 1978; Levy et al., 1977; Loughnan, 1978). In 2 of the studies involving a total of 16 mothers, digoxin was found in breast milk in concentrations of 59 to 75% of that in maternal plasma (Chan et al., 1978; Levy et al., 1977). Loughnan (1978) analysed the plasma of 2 nursing infants whose mothers were taking 0.25mg of digoxin per day. No digoxin could be detected by methods sensitive enough to detect 0.1ng/ml plasma. A more recent study employing a dose of digoxin of 0.75mg daily for seven days could detect the drug in the infant plasma, albeit in small amounts (Finley et al., 1979). Based on these results, on the average milk consumption, and on the average half-life of digoxin in infants, each group of investigators concluded that digoxin would not reach therapeutic plasma concentrations in the nursing infants. The effects of chronic, low dose digoxin administered to infants through breast milk are not known (Chan et al., 1978).

3. Antihypertensive Drugs and Diuretics

Very little is known about the excretion of antihypertensive drugs into breast milk. It has been suggested (Abramowicz, 1974) that reserpine is contraindicated in lactating mothers because of nasal stuffiness, lethargy, and diarrhoea in the nursing infants (Hervada et al., 1978). Supporting data are apparently of an anecdotal nature (Abramowicz, 1979). Propranolol and guanethidine were found in breast milk but no side effects were noted in the nursing infants (Anderson and Salter, 1976; Levitan and Manion, 1973). Based on one mother who received a single 40mg dose of propranolol, Levitan and Manion (1973) calculated that an infant would receive less than, but nearly, a therapeutic dose through mother's milk. Use at a dosage of up to 240mg daily was not associated with untoward effects in a breast-fed infant in another study (Bauer et al, 1979). According to one report, guanethidine appears in breast milk in amounts insufficient to affect the nursing infant, but no details were presented (O'Brien, 1975).

Bendrofluazide, 10mg per day for 5 days, has been used successfully in 40 women to stop lactation (Healy, 1961). This may be the basis for suggestions found in the literature that diuretics can decrease milk production. It has been stated that thrombocytopenia can occur in the infant while the nursing mother is taking chlorothiazide (Abramowicz, 1974). This matter needs documentation. Werthmann and Krees (1972) examined breast milk samples from 11 mothers who took a single 500mg chlorothiazide tablet. Specimens were collected at 1, 2 and 3h after the medication was ingested. The method used could detect $1\mu g/ml$ of chlorothiazide, but the drug was not detected in any of the samples. Based on their data and on known therapeutic blood concentrations, the authors calculated that a nursing infant would receive insignificant quantities of chlorothiazide through the mother's milk and that it should be safe for a nursing mother to use this diuretic. Chlorthalidone has been found in breast milk with a M/P ratio of about 0.03 (Mulley et al., 1978). A ratio of this magnitude is predictable because 98% of the drug is bound to red blood cells at therapeutic plasma concentrations (Dieterle et al., 1976). Even though only a small percentage of the drug is present in milk, Mulley et al. (1978) consider interruption of breast feeding during chlorthalidone therapy important because it has a long half-life (60h) in adults and because pharmacokinetic data are lacking in the neonate.

No data are reported for other antihypertensive drugs.[*]Based on the pH partition concept, a number of antihypertensive drugs, many of which are organic bases, could easily find their way into breast milk and some may even be concentrated there (table XII). Obviously, more studies are needed to determine if the nursing infant will be at risk when the mother takes drugs with effects on the cardiovascular system. Newer and more potent drugs are of special concern.

*Note added in proof: The milk to plasma ratio for captopril was found recently to be quite low (0.012) when the C_{max} in each fluid was compared for 11 subjects. About a 3-fold delay in time to peak level was found for milk with regard to plasma (Devlin and Fleiss, 1980).

11

Gastrointestinal Drugs

John J. Stewart

There are relatively few studies on the pharmacology of the gastrointestinal drugs. Many are found in the older literature and few of the conclusions and hypotheses advanced have been confirmed by workers using modern techniques. Indeed, recent studies have provided a new basis for the classification of laxative agents (Binder, 1977; Gaginella and Bass, 1978), and it would appear that the antacids (Castell and Levine, 1971; Piper and Fenton, 1965) and the narcotic antidiarrhoeal agents (Parolaro et al., 1977; Stewart et al., 1978) have more complex pharmacological mechanisms than originally proposed. Unfortunately, few studies have considered the absorption, distribution, metabolism and excretion of gastrointestinal drugs. It is not surprising, therefore, that little is known about their potential excretion in breast milk.

1. Laxative Agents

Most of the saline cathartics in use today consist of an inorganic salt. Their laxative properties result from the relative nonabsorbability of one of the constituent ions. However, many of these ions have a surprising potential for absorption. Magnesium in ionic form, for example (a popular ingredient in many saline laxative preparations) is approximately 20% absorbed from the gastrointestinal tract (Fingl, 1975). Usually, this absorption is of little consequence in the healthy individual with fully functioning kidneys. Notwithstanding the known absorption of magnesium, much of the literature suggests that saline cathartics containing magnesium and other heavy metal ions can be used safely in the lactating mother (Anderson, 1977; Hervada et al., 1978; Rainbow, 1951). Baldwin's study (1963) went far to foster this attitude. He reported no adverse effects in the nursing infants of mothers given milk of magnesia as a laxative. Whether magnesium appears in the milk after ingesting a laxative containing magnesium has not been determined. Unlikely as this may appear, many would not have predicted its absorption from the gastrointestinal tract and few consider the large quantities of magnesium in a laxative dose of magnesium sulphate. Significant quantities of magnesium in breast milk might be assoiated with diarrhoea, drowsiness, reduced muscle tone and respiratory difficulties in the neonate.

The so-called stimulant cathartics include a heterogeneous group of compounds among which are castor oil, the diphenylmethanes and the anthraquinone laxatives.

Castor oil, a fixed oil pressed from the seeds of *Ricinus communis,* consists of approximately 90 % triricinolein, the triglyceride of ricinoleic acid (Binder et al., 1962). Triricinolein is broken down in the proximal small intestine by the action of pancreatic lipase to form ricinoleic acid, an 18 carbon, unsaturated, hydroxy fatty acid. Ordinarily, the small intestine absorbs long chain fatty acids very efficiently (Wilson, 1962), but large quantities of ricinoleic acid escape absorption and appear in the faeces as soaps of ricinoleic acid or 12-hydroxystearate (Watson and Gordon, 1962; Watson et al., 1963). The unabsorbed ricinoleic acid may reach high intraluminal concentrations throughout the small and large intestine, where it acts locally to inhibit water and electrolyte absorption (Ammon and Phillips, 1973, 1974; Ammon et al., 1974; Bright-Asare and Binder, 1973; Gadacz et al., 1976; Gaginella et al., 1975a,b). The quantity of ricinoleic acid that is absorbed appears to be preferentially distributed to neutral fat rather than phospholipids (Govind Rao et al., 1969; Stewart and Sinclair, 1945).

There are no experimental studies of the concentrations of triricinolein or ricinoleic acid in breast milk and no reports of adverse effects in nursing infants whose mothers had taken a cathartic dose of castor oil. However, when we consider the large quantities of ricinoleic acid absorbed, the possibility of significant concentrations of ricinoleic acid in breast milk becomes more likely. An important factor sometimes overlooked is the quantity of ricinoleic acid present in the average (30g) adult dose of castor oil. Assuming that 90 % of castor oil is triricinolein, and accounting for the glycerol component of the oil, the 30g initial dose of the parent oil would result in the liberation of 24g of ricinoleic acid in the small intestine. If we assume 50 % absorption of ricinoleic acid, an estimate from the clinical data of Watson and Gordon (1962), then 12g of ricinoleic acid would be absorbed. It is difficult to predict whether sufficient levels of triricinolein would appear in breast milk to produce clinically manifest diarrhoea in the infant.

The anthraquinone cathartics consist of several galenical, semipurified and purified preparations. The most popular agents are senna, cascara sagrada, danthron and casanthrol. Cascara sagrada and senna contain many substances, but the active cathartic principles are related chemically to 1,8-dihydroxyanthraquinone or danthron. The anthraquinones in senna and cascara are present as aglycones, glycosides or dianthrone glycosides with glucose and rhamnose as the participating sugar moieties (van Os, 1976). Preparations of cascara sagrada are made from the dried bark of *Rhamnus purshiana* which contains approximately 8 % anthraquinone glycosides and aglycones. Senna is produced either from the leaf or the pod of various species of *Cassia*. Senna varies in its content of anthraquinones, but most sources contain about 2.4 to 4 % of the dianthrone glycosides and sennosides A and B (van Os, 1976). The purified or semipurified preparations, danthron and casanthrol (a mixture of anthranol glycosides extracted from cascara sagrada), are present in many proprietary preparations (Darlington, 1977).

Relatively little is known about the intraintestinal metabolism and absorption of anthraquinone glycosides and aglycones. A thorough review of the subject is presented by van Os (1976a). Because the glycosidic linkages in the anthraquinone glycoside molecules are in the β configuration, little or no hydrolysis occurs in the small intestine of man. The glycosides are not absorbed from the small intestine and pass quantitatively into the colon. The aglycone molecules are at least partially absorbed from the small intestine (Breimer and Baars, 1976) after which they are transported to the liver. Once in the liver, they are glucuronidated and excreted in bile. Since the glucuronidated anthraquinones are not absorbed from the small intestine, they also pass into the colon. In the colon, significant bacterial metabolism of the anthraquinone glycosides and glucuronides occurs, liberating aglycones in the colonic lumen. The aglycones are thought to be absorbed from the colon but to what extent is uncertain.

Since there is significant absorption of aglycone anthraquinones from the small intestine and perhaps from the colon, the agents are potential contaminants of breast milk and a source of adverse effects in the infant. Tyson et al. (1937) found that a number of nursing infants suffered adverse gastrointestinal effects such as diarrhoea and colic when lactating mothers were given cascara sagrada or senna. The authors were only partially successful in documenting the presence of the offending anthraquinone in breast milk in the case of cascara sagrada and completely unsuccessful in the case of senna. Proper controls were not maintained throughout this study and the reliability of the results is questionable. However, Greenleaf and Leonard (1973) also reported a greater incidence of infant diarrhoea when nursing mothers were given senna for postpartum constipation as opposed to other cathartic agents. Still, the presence of anthraquinones in breast milk eludes even relatively modern chemical analytical techniques (Friebel and Walkowiak, 1951).

Most reviewers acknowledge the presence of anthraquinones in breast milk and warn of the consequences for the infant when they are used in the lactating mother

(Bartig and Cohon, 1969; Knowles, 1965, 1974; O'Brien, 1975; Overback, 1974; Vorherr, 1974b). Knowles (1974) and more recently Godding (1976) believe that the anthraquinones have been unjustly maligned in this regard. They ask for more documentation to support the view that the anthraquinones should not be used in lactating mothers.

Phenolphthalein is another cathartic for which the question of excretion into breast milk and adverse effects on the nursing infant is controversial. Tyson et al. (1937) administered 1 grain of phenolphthalein to lactating mothers on the evening of the fifth day after delivery and followed the bowel habits of the infants, as well as the presence of the drug in serial samples of breast milk. 18 of 39 infants were judged to have diarrhoea or colic after mothers received phenolphthalein. However, tests of breast milk in 8 mothers with affected infants failed to show the presence of the drug. Two other studies found no effect on the infant when mothers were given phenolphthalein, nor was phenolphthalein found in breast milk samples (Fantus and Dyniewicz, 1936; Kwit and Hatcher, 1935). Some reviewers conclude that phenolphthalein is not present in human milk and that the drug is not contraindicated in lactating mothers (Bartig and Cohon, 1969; Overbach, 1974; Vorherr, 1974b). Others cite its presence in breast milk but question whether the quantities present are sufficient to cause adverse effects on the infant (Anderson, 1977; Knowles, 1965, 1974; O'Brien, 1975). The differing recommendations reflect the reviewers' interpretation of the clinical data presented in the studies mentioned above.

Bisacodyl is a stimulant cathartic similar to phenolphthalein. Only one reviewer mentions the drug with regard to excretion into breast milk and he states that the drug is not excreted in breast milk (Vorherr, 1974b). However, in making this statement, he offers no documentation. The drug information provided by the manufacturer specifically states that the drug is not contraindicated in lactating mothers, so data establishing the point no doubt exist.

Dioctyl sodium sulphosuccinate (DSS), an anionic surfactant, is often used alone or in combination as a laxative agent. No studies have been performed to determine whether the drug is excreted in breast milk. However, the drug is apparently absorbed. Dujovne and Shoeman (1972) found peak concentrations of DSS of 4 to 9 × 10^{-5}M in bile of adults, 4h after a single oral dose of 100 to 200mg.

The emollient laxative, mineral oil, is a mixture of liquid hydrocarbons obtained from petroleum. Although the drug is generally considered 'indigestible', at least a slight absorption is indicated by visualisation of the oil in the mesenteric lymph nodes, spleen and liver of chronic users (Fingl, 1975). The drug probably would not appear in breast milk.

The bulk forming agents consist of a number of natural or partially purified polysaccharides and cellulose-like compounds derived mainly from plant sources. Little intestinal metabolism occurs in man because of a lack of the appropriate glucosidase. Agents like bran, plantago ovata coating and psyllium hydrophyllic mucilloid are probably the laxatives of choice for the lactating mother.

2. Antiulcer Agents

The antacids possess a potential for excretion in breast milk at least equal to that of the saline cathartics. In many cases, the antacids and the saline cathartics contain the same inorganic active ingredients, but the antacid preparations rely more heavily upon combinations of inorganic salts.

The antacids are often identified as systemic or nonsystemic, based upon their relative absorption from the gut. A systemic antacid, like sodium bicarbonate, adds to the total intraintestinal bicarbonate pool and absorption of bicarbonate occurs. The body excretes the excess bicarbonate to maintain acid-base balance and in the process excretory fluids like urine and perhaps breast milk are alkalinised. The effects of bicarbonate ingestion on breast milk composition or pH have not been studied. The use of sodium bicarbonate as an antacid should be discouraged in all patients.

The nonsystemic antacids, like calcium carbonate and magnesium and aluminium oxides and hydroxides, are relatively nonabsorbed. The titration of gastric acid by a nonsystemic antacid is accompanied by regeneration of an insoluble, relatively nonabsorbed salt in the small intestine. Alteration of acid-base balance is not a major concern with nonsystemic antacid therapy. Toxic effects produced by the significant absorption of the cationic species or their effects on the absorption and body stores of other ions are of greater importance. Increased maternal plasma concentrations of ions like magnesium and aluminium are a source of concern, particularly in view of the significant gastrointestinal absorption of magnesium (Fingl, 1976) and aluminium (Schroeder and Nason, 1971) ions which is known to occur. Plasma or breast milk concentrations of magnesium or aluminium after administration of antacid doses of magnesium or aluminium salts have not been studied.

Preparations containing belladonna alkaloids may be prescribed for the treatment of peptic ulcer. The major alkaloid found in belladonna, atropine, is well absorbed from the gastrointestinal tract and widely distributed in the body. Atropine is sometimes said to be contraindicated in lactating mothers for 2 reasons: it is excreted in human milk and may produce toxic signs and symptoms in the infant, and secondly it decreases the production of breast milk (Anderson, 1977; Arena, 1966; O'Brien, 1975). Both these statements have been challenged. Some authors specifically state that atropine is not excreted in breast milk (Illingworth, 1953; Knowles, 1965; Overbach, 1974), or that the drug does not reach significant concentrations in breast milk to affect the nursing infant (Vorherr, 1974b). Atropine has also been said not to affect the quantity of breast milk produced (Innes and Nickerson, 1975). It appears that there is no good documentation of either objection to the use of atropine in lactating mothers. However, because of the particular sensitivity of infants to anticholinergic agents (Unna et al., 1950), a prudent action would be to avoid atropine-containing preparations in the lactating mother.

The quaternary ammonium anticholinergic agents such as glycopyrronium (glycopyrrolate), oxyphenonium, isopropramide, mepenzolate and propantheline are synthetic drugs which have been used as antiulcer and antispasmodic medications. Little is known about their distribution and excretion but because they are charged compounds at physiological pH, one would expect little, if any, to gain entrance to human milk. However, the question of their excretion in breast milk has not as yet been answered by carefully performed clinical studies.

Currently, cimetidine is enjoying wide use as an antiulcer agent. Although a recent review stated that the drug is excreted in human breast milk (Clayman, 1977), documentation of its presence in breast milk is apparently lacking (Karpow et al., 1978). Recently, however, a M/P ratio of 5 to 12 was shown for one patient (Somogyi and Gugler, 1979). Generally, it is recommended that cimetidine not be given during lactation.

3. Antidiarrhoeal Agents

The antidiarrhoeal agents consist of: adsorbents, anticholinergics, galenical preparations containing opium powder, and the newer synthetic, morphine-like compounds with greatly reduced central actions. Morphine and morphine-like drugs are generally regarded as the most effective antidiarrhoeal agents.

The most popular adsorbents consist of various hydrated aluminium and magnesium-aluminium silicates or clays (e.g. kaolin and attapulgite), bismuth salts, pectin and charcoal. For the most part, these compounds are not known to be absorbed from the gastrointestinal tract. Even the clays, which contain potentially toxic ions, are apparently insufficiently soluble for much absorption to occur. Generally, these preparations are probably safe to use in the lactating mother.

The use of anticholinergic agents in the lactating mother is often regarded as unsafe, as mentioned previously. Because of their questionable effectiveness in many diarrhoeal patients and the question of their excretion in breast milk, another more generally effective and safer antidiarrhoeal preparation should be used.

Morphine is an effective antidiarrhoeal agent in relatively low doses. When morphine is used as an antidiarrhoeal agent, it is usually provided in the form of paregoric, a hydroalcoholic solution containing opium powder. Paregoric contains enough opium powder to provide approximately 2mg of morphine base in the usual adult dose. This quantity of morphine is far below the clinical dose administered for analgesia. The general consensus is that morphine is excreted in human milk but that the concentrations present are clinically insignificant (Arena, 1966; Bartig and Cohon, 1969; Kwit and Hatcher, 1935; O'Brien, 1975). However, there are remarkably few studies in which the presence and quantity of morphine in human milk have been tested. Terwilliger and Hatcher (1934) found no drug present in the breast milk of mothers receiving 128mg of morphine sulphate daily. Anderson (1977) cites 2 cases in which 16mg of morphine given parenterally was accompanied by undetectable concentrations of drug in breast milk in 1 case, and less than 6µg/ml in another.

Observations of narcotic-addicted mothers who were nursing infants suggest strongly that some opiates appear in breast milk in significant quantities. Weaning infants of addicted mothers is often accompanied by opiate withdrawal symptoms in the child (Cobrinik et al., 1959). It should be emphasised, however, that careful pharmacokinetic studies of morphine concentrations in breast milk have not been performed.

Diphenoxylate is a potent antidiarrhoeal agent which apparently acts on opiate receptors to produce antidiarrhoeal effects. The compound is said to be almost devoid of central morphine-like actions, except in exceptionally high doses. The drug is marketed in combination with a subtherapeutic dose of atropine (25µg per adult dosage unit) which is included in the preparation to discourage abuse. The only information available on its presence in breast milk is contained in the drug information literature provided by the manufacturer which warns of the drug's presence in human milk. A similar agent, loperamide, seems to have even less central action than diphenoxylate. It is not known whether loperamide appears in human breast milk in sufficient quantities to affect the nursing infant. Neither drug should be used in the lactating mother.

12

Insecticides, Pollutants and Toxins

Barbara R. Manno

Of the many environmental agents to which humans are exposed, only a few have been found in human milk (table XIII). More have been demonstrated in the milk of ruminants and other non-ruminant animals, but with a few exceptions these will not be considered here. The absence of reports on environmental agents results primarily from a failure to relate a sick breast-fed infant to exposure of the mother to an environmental toxicant. In addition, testing procedures in the past may have been lacking or insufficiently sensitive to detect the actual presence of the toxicant (see section 5).

Pharmacokinetic interpretations for this broad group of chemical agents rely heavily on existing knowledge for compounds with similar physical and chemical properties as well as the current state of knowledge in regard to basic mechanisms proposed for transport across the blood-milk barrier and subsequent appearance of the agent in the milk (see section 4). Milk analysis for environmental pollutants, however, must be carefully evaluated to ensure that external contamination of the specimens has not occurred. This caveat is emphasised by studies of bacteria and virus contamination of milk (Anderson, 1977; Knowles, 1965, 1974; Vorherr, 1974b).

Olszyna-Marzys (1978) has classified environmental toxic agents into two categories: social and ecological toxicants. The former category represents those toxic agents whose intake man can control, such as nicotine and ethanol. Reports of nicotine in the milk of mothers who smoke are conflicting. However, more recent work indicates that smoking 20 to 30 cigarettes per day may produce low concentra-

Table XIII. Environmental agents identified in human milk

Agent	Reference
Herbicide Kerb	St. John and Lisk (1975)
Lipid-soluble chlorinated hydro-carbons DDT DDE DDD Heptachlor epoxide HCB PCB Dieldrin Aldrin Mirex Hexachlorobenzene Lindane Parathion Paroxon	Bagnell and Ellenberger (1977); Bakken and Seip (1976); Bond and Woodham (1975); Curley and Kimbrough (1969); Dyment et al. (1971a,b); Hagyard et al. (1973); Hawthorne et al. (1974); Hayes (1976); Hornabrook et al. (1972); Jan et al. (1975); Kojima and Araki (1975); Kroger (1972); Luquet et al. (1972, 1975); Masuda et al. (1974); Mes et al. (1978); Musial et al. (1974); Olszyma-Marzys (1978); Pesendorfer (1975); Pfielsticker (1973); Quinby (1965); Risebrough (1969); Savage et al. (1973); Siyali (1973); Vaori et al. (1977); Wilson et al. (1973); Winter et al. (1976); Woodard (1976).
Nicotine	Catz and Giacola (1972); Illingworth (1953); Perlman et al. (1942).
Immunological factors	Beer and Billingham (1975); Jelliffe and Jelliffe (1977).
Metal ions Mercury Iron Zinc Selenium Cadmium Lead	Amin-Zaki et al. (1974a); Amin-Zaki et al. (1974b); Amin-Zaki et al. (1976); Fujita et al. (1977); Garcia et al. (1974); Glenn and Hamsard (1964); Ladinskaya et al. (1973); Levin et al. (1976); Lombek et al. (1978); McClanahan et al. (1965); Neathery and Miller (1975); Schulte-Lobbert et al. (1977).
Miscellaneous ^{137}Cesium ^{210}Lead ^{210}Polonium ^{129}Iodine Iodine Bromide	Daly et al. (1974); Gustafson and Miller (1969); Klemmer et al. (1977); Pendleton and Lloyd (1974); Stewart and Vidor (1976).

tions of nicotine in the milk (Ferguson et al., 1976). Strict adherence to the two classes of toxicants, social and ecological, found in milk does not permit inclusion of endogenous toxins from the maternal metabolism which may be excreted in milk. These would include intermediates of incomplete maternal carbohydrate metabolism as seen in avitaminosis B_1 (beriberi). These intermediates are lactic acid, acetoacetic

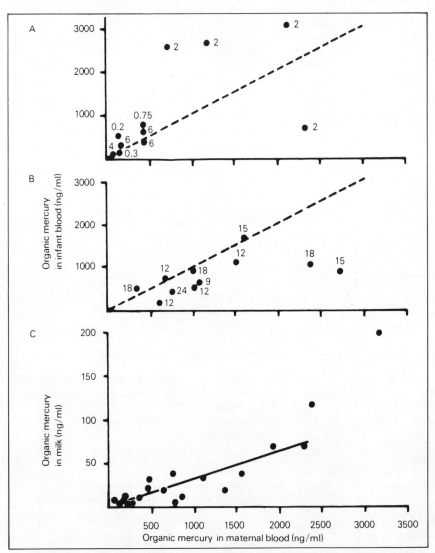

Fig. 19. The relationship between concentrations of organic mercury in the blood of infants and in maternal milk and the concentration of organic mercury in samples of maternal blood. A) Blood samples from infants who were born during and after the epidemic and were thus exposed to methyl mercury *in utero* and in maternal milk. B) Blood samples from infants who were born prior to the epidemic and were thus exposed only to methyl mercury in maternal milk. C) Samples of maternal milk collected at intervals between April and July, 1972.

The number adjacent to the points in A and B indicate the age of the infant in months at the time of sampling. The dotted lines in A and B are lines of equality. The line in C is the linear regression line calculated from the mercury concentrations in maternal blood that were below 2500ng/ml (Bakir et al., 1973).

acid, glucuronic acid, methylglyoxal and pyruvic acid (Fehily, 1944; Knowles, 1974). These chemicals are not within the scope of this review.

Primary considerations influencing excretion of environmental agents in milk include the plasma-milk pH differential, plasma protein binding of the toxic agent, molecular weight of the compound, the polarity of the agent and its lipids and water-solubility (see section 4). Other factors which may directly alter transport and excretion of the particular agent also include the dose of the agent, duration of exposure, single or multiple exposure, route of exposure, urban or rural environment, seasonal variation of exposure and species studied.

The most extensively reported environmental exposures have involved chlorinated hydrocarbon compounds (Olszyna-Marzys, 1978; Winter et al., 1976), e.g. hexachlorobenzene, dicophane or DDT [1,1,1-trichloro-2,2-bis(p-chlorophenyl) ethanel] and its analogues and metabolites, polychlorinated biphenyls (Masuda et al., 1974), and organic mercurial compounds such as methyl mercury (Amin-Zaki et al., 1974a,b, 1976; Fujita and Takabutake, 1977). These reports were derived from exposure of people in sufficient number to provide both the impetus and population for study.

In general, lactating animals are not routinely included when studies are performed to ascertain absorption, distribution and excretion of a chemical agent. Most milk excretion studies, however, are conducted in lactating ruminants. The problem of extrapolation of data from ruminants (bovine) to humans becomes evident when the literature on the lipid-soluble insecticides is evaluated. Man excreted 125% of daily intake while the cow excreted only 1.5% of its daily intake of DDT (Knowles, 1974). The majority of human DDT citations are epidemiological in nature. However, it has been demonstrated that DDT can promote its own increased excretion. After demonstrating the lack of Mirex elimination in milk, it was postulated that 'something' occurs which may alter the agent during digestion in the ruminant (Bond and Woodham, 1975). Route of administration may then be a very important determinant for finding Mirex and other lipid-soluble chemicals in milk.

The hepatic microsomal enzyme metabolism of dieldrin in animals and man is altered by the presence of other lipid-soluble pesticides, such as DDT (Alary et al., 1971; Conneyn 1967; Cueto and Hayes, 1965; Durham, 1969; Fries et al., 1971; Klemmer et al., 1977; Shimada and Ugawa, 1978; Street, 1964; Street et al., 1966). Drugs such as phenobarbitone, phenylbutazone, tolbutamide, aminopyrine, and heptabarbitone have been shown to decrease tissue (lipid) stores of lipid-soluble insecticides (Street et al., 1966). Phenytoin decreased milk concentration of DDT, DDE [1,1-dichloro-2,2-bis(p-chlorophenyl) ethylene] and DDD [1,1-dichloro-2,2-bis(p-chlorophenyl)ethane] (Fries et al., 1971). These collective findings should help to explain the excretion of DDT and other lipid-soluble insecticides in excess of daily intake in man. It is therefore important to consider what exposure of nursing mothers to other environmental agents and drugs which alter hepatic microsomal enzyme metabolism is clinically relevant if simultaneous exposure to lipid-soluble toxicants occurs. Little has been added since the reviews of Hayes (1965), Conney (1967) and Durham (1969) to define the pharmacokinetics of the pesticides in the mammalian system.

Few studies have evaluated the postpartum interval used for human milk collection and subsequent toxicant or natural component analysis (see section 3). During the first week postpartum, more water-soluble compounds may be present in colostrum. Excretion of such compounds as lead, zinc, selenium, iron and cadmium in colostrum is greater than in mature milk (Daly et al., 1974; Ladinskaya et al., 1973; Gustafson and Miller, 1969; Pendleton and Lloyd, 1974; Stewart and Vidor, 1976).

Methyl mercury poisoning occurred in a major portion of the population of Iraq in late 1971 and early 1972. This resulted from ingestion of bread made from contaminated grain. Data from this unfortunate experience are the basis for a comprehensive study (Amin-Zaki et al., 1974a,b, 1976; Bakir et al., 1973). Three rele-

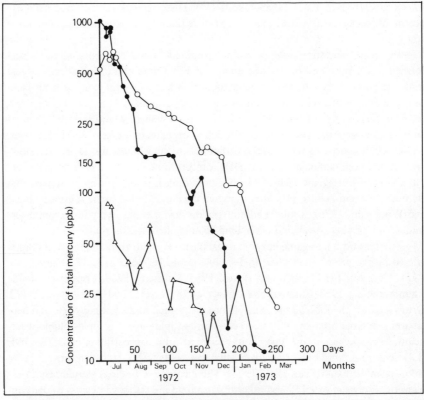

Fig. 20. Concentration of total mercury in infant's blood and in mother's blood and milk. The date of birth was June, 1971 (Amin-Zaki et al., 1974b).
○ Infant's blood ● Maternal blood △ Milk.

vant population subgroups of fetal and infant poisoning were identified: (a) infants exposed to methyl mercury solely via maternal milk; (b) infants exposed *in utero* and subsequently via maternal milk; and (c) infants who may have been exposed *in utero*. It was possible to correlate mercury concentrations in maternal blood with those in milk and in infant blood, and these were compared with length of exposure and clinical symptomatology (fig. 19) [Amin-Zaki et al., 1974a,b; Bakir et al., 1973). Bakir et al. (1973) demonstrated that, in those infants exposed *in utero* and during nursing, the blood mercury concentration was slightly higher than that of maternal blood. The milk concentration was about 3% of maternal blood concentrations. Amin-Zaki et al. (1974a,b) found a decline of methyl mercury in infant and maternal blood for a period of 250 days of breast feeding (fig. 20). However, for several infants the ratio of infant to maternal blood concentrations increased during a similar period of breast feeding. There is no explanation for a higher ratio at lower blood concentrations.

While most calculations of previous human exposure have been related to experimental models weighing 70kg, the Iraq exposure involved a population of much smaller weight (51kg average). 34% of the exposed population comprised children of different ages. Maternal blood mercury concentration was found to be more predictive of the extent of exposure than was the urine mercury level (Bakir et al., 1973). Given these collective observations on total body burden, it is apparent that correlations between current findings (Amin-Zaki et al., 1974a,b, 1976; Bakir et al., 1973) and previously cited works would be difficult since populations with disparate characteristics are described.

While investigations such as those from Iraq and others (see also Kroger, 1974) cannot be planned well in advance of their occurrence, many improved approaches to design can be gained from retrospective analysis. Proper planning enables rapid initiation of large scale epidemiological, laboratory and clinical studies once the 'chance' observation identifies an environmental toxin exposure of an extensive nature. The literature should be scanned to update procedural design to complete gaps in our knowledge regarding the disposition and clinical effects of environmental toxins, especially on breast feeding infants. Lack of a plan of study has minimised the collection of available data, even when the opportunity presented itself.

13

Milk/Plasma Ratios and Contraindicated Drugs

John T. Wilson

Table XIV lists the observed M/P ratio of drugs for which milk and plasma concentration data are available in man. The observed M/P ratio for whole milk is often less than that predicted by ion partitioning in an ultrafiltrate of milk and plasma. This probably results from water displacement by fat and protein (see section 3). It should be recalled that the majority of M/P ratios need additional information on drug dosing in relation to the pattern of breast feeding. Most data are derived from reports of single case histories and are not based on AUC comparisons for a drug in milk and plasma. Nevertheless, special concern should be given to those drugs which have a M/P $>$ 1(Shirkey, 1980).

Analysis of this list (Vorherr, 1974a,b) revealed that the infant would receive only 5 drugs [(chloramphenicol, phenytoin, radioactive iodine (^{131}I), phenobarbitone and thiouracil] in more than 1 % of the total daily maternal dose. This is consistent with a more recent review (Abramowicz, 1979) which listed antithyroid drugs (see below), radioactive iodine, lithium, chloramphenicol and most anticancer drugs as definitely contraindicated with regard to risk for the breast feeding infant.

Others (Hervada et al., 1978) have cited chloramphenicol, metronidazole, propylthiouracil, radioactive isotopes, tetracycline, ergot alkaloids, and iodides as being contraindicated in women who are breast feeding. There is only one report relating to concentration of antithyroid drugs in breast milk and that relates to thiouracil (Williams et al., 1944). No specific data are available for any of the antithyroid drugs currently used and presumably findings with thiouracil have been extrapolated to the other drugs*. Regrettably data on the physicochemical or pharmacokinetic properties of these agents are not available to enable us to know whether such extrapolation is

---

Note added in proof: Kampman et al. (1980) present data on propylthiouracil and suggest that the drug may be used cautiously in breast feeding women if the thyroid status of the infant is carefully monitored.

Table XIV. Human milk to plasma ratio (M/P) for various drugs

Drug	M/P[1]		
Aspirin	0.6-1	Isoniazid	1.0
Bishydroxycoumarin (dicoumarol)	0.01-0.02	Kanamycin sulphate	0.05-0.40
Bis 3: 3-4 oxycoumarinylethylacetate	0.6-0.8[b]	Lincomycin	0.13-0.17
Carbamazepine	0.6-07[c]	Lithium carbonate	0.35-0.36
Chloral hydrate	0-0.50	Meprobamate	2-4[a]
	0.27[b]	Methotrexate	0.10
Chloramphenicol	0.50-0.60	Metronidazole	0.6-1.4[c]
	0.05[b]	Nalidixic acid	0.08-0.13
Chlorpromazine	0.3	d-Norgestrel	0.2
	0.5[b]	Novobiocin	0.10-0.25
Colistin sulphate	0.17-0.18	Penicillin	0.03-0.20
			0.02-0.2[b]
Cycloserine	0.67-0.75	Phenobarbitone	0.17-0.28
Desmethyldiazepam	0.1[c]	Pentothal	1.0[b]
Diazepam	0.1[c]	Phenytoin	0.4-2.0
Dihydroxystreptomycin	0.02-0.1[b]	Phenylbutazone	0.10-0.12
Digoxin	0.8-0.9[c]		0.10-0.30[c]
Epoxycarbamazepine	0.6-1.0[c]	Propylthiouracil	12[a]
		Pyrazolone	1.0[b]
		Pyrimethamine	0.20-0.43
Erythromycin	2.5-3.0	Quinine sulphate	0.14
	0.5[b]	Rifampicin (rifampin)	0.20-0.60
Ethanol	1.0	Streptomycin sulphate	0.50-1.0
Ether	1.0[b]	Sulphatrone	6.4[b]
Ethyl biscoumacetate	0-0.01	Sulphapyridine	1.0
Folic acid	0.02	Sulphanilamide	1.0[a]
		Tetracycline hydrochloride	0.62-0.81
Flufenamic acid	< 0.01[c]		0.25-1.5[b]
Imipramine hydrochloride	0.08-0.50	Thiouracil	3
Iodine 131	65	Tolbutamide	0.25[a]

1   The M/P ratio is shown for milk to maternal plasma.
  Data calculated from that cited by Vorherr (1974a,b) for milk and plasma drug concentrations and from M/P ratios quoted by: a = Hervada (1978); b = Knowles (1972) and c = Shirkey (1980).

reasonable or not. Adverse clinical effects in breast feeding neonates have not been described. Cautionary statements (Hervada et al., 1978) were given for yet other drugs (nalidixic acid, sulphonamides, antimalarials, isoniazid, meprobamate, lithium, phenytoin, primidone, chronically administered salicylates, atropine, and caffeine). Gastrointestinal drugs such as diphenoxylate, loperamide and cimetidine should probably be added to a list of prescribed agents. Drug combinations with potential for adverse effects would include the methylxanthines and respiratory depressants (ethanol, narcotics, barbiturates). As emphasised repeatedly in this review, additional studies are needed to either substantiate contraindications or obviate these restrictions.

While the expected infant dose of most drugs from breast milk is not large, 13% of drugs in the 1973 Physician's Desk Reference (USA) were proscribed for breast feeding women (Wilson, 1975) generally from lack of information. The majority of drugs, while not actually proscribed, are given with unknown risk to the breast feeding infant, again, from lack of information.

14

Consequences of Breast Milk Drug Dosing on Infant Behaviour and Development

D.R. Cherek

Limited research reports of the behaviour of offspring following drugs administered to breast feeding mothers have appeared. Two reports have demonstrated that drugs administered to lactating animals can affect motor activity of the offspring. Lundborg (1972) found that haloperidol (1 mg/kg/day) administered to nursing rabbit dams resulted in motor impairment of the offspring, a marked inability to elevate themselves, difficulty in head raising and lack of coordination of the hind limbs. Haloperidol administered in equivalent parenteral doses to young rabbits (who were not exposed to the drug during nursing) did not result in the same motor impairments. In a more recent study, Buckalew (1978) found that administration of a 5% solution of ethanol to lactating mice resulted in a decrement in motor activity when compared with the offspring of mice who were not exposed to ethanol in the mother's milk.

Ahlenius et al., (1973, 1975, 1977) in a series of studies investigated the offspring's behaviour after administering 2 antipsychotic drugs (penfluridol and pimozide) to nursing rat dams. In their initial study (Ahlenius et al., 1973), nursing rat dams were administered 1 mg/kg of penfluridol on days 1, 3 and 5 after delivery. Then the male littermates were tested for acquisition of a conditioned avoidance response 4 weeks after birth. The behavioural task consisted of discrete avoidance trials utilising a 2-way shuttle box. The sound of a buzzer (the conditioned stimulus) was presented for 10 seconds. At the end of 10 seconds, intermittent shock (the unconditioned stimulus) was delivered through the grid floor of either compartment.

The behavioural measures were:

1) A conditioned avoidance response, i.e. the rat crossing the opening from one chamber to the other within the 10 seconds after the buzzer was presented, and (2)

2) Escape response, crossing to the other side of the compartment within 10 seconds of the shock being delivered.

Offspring of mothers administered glucose during nursing started with 75% of their responses being conditioned avoidance responses and reached 100% avoidance responses (i.e. avoiding all the shocks) after the third training session. Offsprings of dams given penfluridol during nursing showed initial avoidance responses of 35% of the total responses, and they reached the level of 90% avoidance responses only after the fifth session. Thus, there was an overall retardant effect of penfluridol on the acquisition of this conditioned avoidance response. Interestingly, there was no disruption of escape responses in either group so that the administration of penfluridol during nursing influenced only the conditioned avoidance response.

Further studies with penfluridol (1mg/kg/day) were undertaken to assess the effect on gross motor activity and open field behaviour in the offspring (Ahlenius et al., 1977). Again penfluridol was administered on days 1, 3, 5, and 7 after delivery and the offspring were investigated at 6 to 18 days of age to assess their motor behaviour development. No differences were found between glucose control and penfluridol offspring with regard to movement of the head and/or forelegs, walking, and startle response to an auditory stimulus. At 4 weeks of age the penfluridol and glucose control treated offspring were tested in an open field maze. At 4 weeks of age the penfluridol treated offspring displayed higher locomotor activity than the controls. At 8 and 12 weeks of age the glucose control treated offspring had increased their level of activity markedly. However, the penfluridol treated offspring showed a decrease in activity to a level lower than the controls. This is in contrast to the normal rat behaviour which shows an increase in open field activity with increasing age. The higher activity and lower defaecation scores shown by the 4-week-old penfluridol treated offspring suggest a lowered 'emotional reactivity' in these animals. The relatively low reactivity to stimuli may contribute to the impaired acquisition of an active avoidance response seen in the previous study.

Ahlenius et al. (1975) also investigated the behavioural effects in offspring after administration of pimozide (0.5mg/kg/day) to nursing rat dams on 7 consecutive days after delivery. Utilising the same discrete shock avoidance task in a 2-way shuttle box, they again observed a similar deficit in acquisition of the conditioned avoidance response in offspring exposed to pimozide in the mother's milk.

To investigate the possible basis of this observed decrement in acquisition of a conditioned avoidance response, these investigators analysed the concentration and turnover of neurotransmitters in regional brain areas of offspring from mothers treated with the same dose of penfluridol (Engel and Lundborg, 1974). They found that the offspring from mothers treated with penfluridol showed a marked decrease in the rate of tyrosine hydrosylation in specific brain regions. They also found that the levels of noradrenaline (norepinephrine) were significantly decreased in the limbic system, brain stem and diencephalon. The 5-HT concentration was also decreased in the hemispheres. They concluded that penfluridol possibly interacts with the development of brain monoamine mechanisms at sensitive developmental periods. This interaction thereby induces a decreased functional activity in central monoamine neurons, especially in the limbic system, and a consequent effect on the acquisition of conditioned avoidance responses is observed.

The pimozide induced deficit in conditioned avoidance response as observed in a 2-way shuttle box task (with and without visual cues or stimuli) could be reversed following the administration of d-amphetamine (0.5 and 2.0mg/kg). Thus, the administration of d-amphetamine to offspring of rat dams treated with pimozide resulted in a marked increase in conditioned avoidance responses as compared with poor performance of saline treated offspring of mothers treated with pimozide. The d-amphetamine did not produce a general increase in all responses, since in the visual discrimination avoidance task, only the correct responses were increased and not the level of incorrect avoidance responses. The observed behavioural deficits in the offspring of nursing mothers treated with antipsychotics were apparently due to developmental disturbances in central catecholamine neurons. Amphetamine is able to reverse this behavioural deficit by increasing the activity of central catecholamine neurons.

A few investigators have examined offspring behaviour following administration of lead to nursing mothers. Sauerhoff and Michaelson (1973) found that offspring of nursing rat dams eating a diet containing 4% lead carbonate displayed excessive stereotyped behaviour manifested by excessive self-grooming which started at 4 weeks of age. These offspring also had a 40 to 90% increase in spontaenous motor activity as measured by a Selective Activity Metre. Snowdon (1973) found that when rat dams were injected with lead acetate (0.8mg/100g of body weight) throughout lactation, their offspring developed more slowly, weighed less and demonstrated performance deficits on a Hegg Williams maze for food reinforcement. The offspring of lead treated mothers committed more errors in the maze and took more sessions to reach performance criteria. The authors concluded that the effects were not due to a general motor activity deficit or augmentation since there were no differences in running times between offspring of lead and non-lead treated mothers. Brown (1975) investigated the effects of lead acetate, administered to nursing dams in drinking water (10mg/100ml) or by oral administration (25-35mg/kg/day), on offsping behaviour. The dams were treated with lead for the total nursing period of 21 days and the offspring were tested at 8 to 10 weeks of age. Offspring from lead treated dams and vehicle treated dams did not differ in the level of spontaneous motor activity or in open field maze behaviour (i.e. measurement of number of grids crossed, number of faecal boli and number of rearings). Offspring were also tested in a T-maze for water reinforcement. This was a discrimination task such that when the runway was illuminated, the water was in the left arm of the maze and when the light was off, the water was in the right arm of the maze. The offspring of mothers who were administered lead acetate showed a performance deficit in the T-maze. Offspring whose mothers ingested lead acetate in the drinking water (average consumption of 17.5mg/kg/day) averaged 3.8 successes (i.e., at least 5 correct responses on 6 consecutive trials) compared to an average of 8.0 for vehicle-treated offspring. Offspring of mothers given oral doses of lead acetate (25-35mg/kg/day) averaged 2.7 successes compared with 4.2 for the control offspring. This study demonstrated that a performance or behavioural deficit was produced by low doses of lead which did not result in overt signs of lead toxicity, altered liver, body or brain weights, increased brain water content or changes in spontaneous motor activity or exploratory behaviour. Only the T-maze water-reinforced task was sensitive enough to detect the behavioural toxicity induced by the lead.

In reviewing the research reports cited above, as well as others, one must consider problems of research design. Three aspects of studies require attention:

1) Assignment of offspring to treatment groups
2) Techniques of administering drugs to the lactating dams
3) Selection of behavioural tasks.

Early studies simply assigned the nursing mothers to drug or vehicle treatment groups and thus the genetic variability of offspring from different litters was not considered. In later studies, the young from several litters were mixed at birth and assigned at random to different dams. The dams in turn were assigned at random to drug or vehicle treatment. In an attempt to reduce the variability between groups of offspring, cross-fostering appears to be the best technique. Littermates should be assigned to drug and vehicle treated dams for nursing, so that there are equal numbers of littermates in the vehicle group and drug treatment groups (if more than one dose is used). Thus, equivalent proportions of the litters would be composed of offspring assigned to their biological dam and of offspring assigned to their non-biological dam. This procedure is an attempt to distribute the intra-litter genetic variability throughout the different treatment groups. The technique of cross-fostering has been found to exert no effect on the performance in a 2-way shuttle box avoidance task (Gauron and Rowley, 1973).

Lundborg (1972), Buckalew (1978) and Sauerhoff and Michaelson (1973) administered the drugs in the drinking water or food of the nursing mother. The lack of control when these methods are used favours the administration of drugs orally to the nursing dam. Oral dosing provides for an accurate amount of drug and intervals between doses which are necessary for adequate control of drug exposure. Dose response determinations are conspicuously absent from these studies; only one dose of the drug was studied. The use of more than one dose of the drug necessitates the use of at least one litter for each drug dosage. This adds to the size of the experiments, but strengthens the relationship between the observed behavioural effect in the offspring and the drug administered to the dam.

In selecting behavioural baselines to assess effects on offspring behaviour, one is faced with the major problem of studying and assessing an irreversible drug treatment effect. Therefore, the numerous operant conditioning procedures which utilise the subject as his own control cannot be employed and one is faced with the major problem of studying and assessing an irreversible drug treatment effect. Instead one is forced to utilise group studies with the inherent intersubject variability that these studies entail (Burt, 1975; Sidman, 1960). This is particularly true of experiments concerned with the effects of drugs on development as illustrated by the present studies, since no meaningful pretreatment performance data can be obtained. Initial observations of body movement and spontaneous activity may be useful in detecting gross motor effects of the drugs. Utilisation of discrete conditioned shock avoidance tasks (such as the 2-way shuttle box) is an advantage because one can measure the effects of drugs on escape as well as avoidance responses to determine the specificity of drug effect in terms of a general depressive or excitatory effect on all behaviour. Differential effects of many drugs on avoidance behaviour as opposed to escape behaviour have long been recognised (Dews and Morse, 1961). Discrete trial, discriminated shock avoidance techniques can be used where bar pressing responses are utilised instead of crossing over a shuttle box. One technique which has been used to assess behavioural toxicity of drugs has been a DRL food reinforcement schedule, in which subjects are reinforced for lever pressing, only when they space their responses by at least a specified time interval (Sidman, 1959). For a more complete discussion of behavioural baselines with which to assess behavioural toxicity, the reader is referred to the book 'Behavioral Toxicology' by Weiss and Laties (1975).

Most infant behaviour studies involving drugs in breast milk are restricted to experimental animals because of ethical considerations. In man, some gross behavioural observations, such as lethargy and impaired suckling, were found in breast-fed infants of mothers receiving drugs such as diazepam (Mirkin, 1976). Stechler (1964) attempted to assess behavioural toxicity in 2- to 4-day-old neonates exposed to various drugs during delivery. He assessed attentive behaviour by measuring time spent viewing a card or cards containing pictures of a die or face. Techniques such as these, together with operant conditioning techniques may be used to assess behavioural effects in neonates whose nursing mothers received medication during their first few days of life. Most drugs are excreted in human milk in small quantities, and consequent gross anatomical and motor side effects are often not apparent. Subtle behavioural problems may develop, however, and they may remain covert until testing techniques or psychosocial stresses uncover the lesion.

r.

15

Conclusions

John T. Wilson

Concern about infant dosing of drugs via breast milk will increase in direct proportion to the prevalence of breast feeding, maternal drug consumption, and to our lack of knowledge about both the amount of drug in milk and its associated risks. This review reveals the paucity of information to be found on all aspects of the subject in humans.

The present understanding of breast milk excretion processes and milk composition changes should enable a more comprehensive approach to the collection of pharmacological data. Predictions about the amount of drug in milk can be derived from drug and tissue fluid characteristics. Measurements of drug in milk can be made in a relevant and pharmacokinetic manner to test these predictions. The proposed infant-modulated 3-compartment open model for drug disposition in lactating women can be evaluated by the analysis of drug in plasma and milk over an extended period after dosing. As proposed, data consistent with a deep third compartment (i.e. breast milk) would greatly facilitate a pharmacokinetic modeling approach aimed at the assessment of milk concentrations in regard to time of dosing and breast feeding.

Long term consequences may occur in the infant who is chronically dosed with a drug via breast milk. Subtle behavioural changes, as one consequence, may be manifested only when pubertal or adult psychosocial stresses uncover the hitherto covert lesion. Growth and biochemical disturbances may be more immediate and evident.

The human lactating female and her infant are clearly the most suitable subjects for the required studies on drug excretion in breast milk. Given the appropriate medical and ethical setting, these subjects can provide samples for drug analysis and, with the proper pharmacokinetic approach, provide data most applicable to their health care needs. Funding sources for such studies must recognise the opportunistic nature of the investigation. Sufficient and protracted sources are needed if accurate data are to be obtained. Analytical, pharmacokinetic and biological approaches are now ready to go beyond the single case study in order to develop guiding principles in this most important area of infant nutrition and paediatric clinical pharmacology.

References

Aaes-Jorgensen, T. and Jorgensen, A.: Studies of excretion in rabbit milk after administration of car-
bon-14 labelled amitriptyline and nortriptyline. Archives Internationales de Pharmacodynamie et de
Therapie 227: 294-301 (1977).

Abramowicz, M. (Ed): Drugs in Breast Milk. Medical Letter 16: 25-27 (1974).

Abramowicz, M. (Ed) Update: Drugs in Breast Milk. Medical Letter 21: 21-24 (1979).

Addy, H.A.: The breast feeding of twins: An exploratory study. Journal of Tropical Pediatric and Environmental Child Health 21: 231 (1975).

Ahlenius, S.; Brown, R.; Engel, J. and Lundborg, P.: Learning deficits in 4 week old offspring of the
nursing mothers treated with the neuroleptic drug penfluridol. Naunyn-Schmiedeberg's Archives of
Pharmacology 279: 31.37 (1973).

Ahlenius, S.; Engel, J. and Lundborg, P.: Antagonism by d-emphetamine of learning deficits in rats induced by exposure to antipsychotic drugs during postnatal life. Naunyn-Schmiedeberg's Archives of
Pharmacology 288: 185-193 (1975).

Ahlenius, S.; Engel, J.; Hard, E.; Larsson, K.; Lundborg, P. and Sinnerstedt, P.: Open field behaviour and
gross motor development in offspring of nursing rat mothers given penfluridol. Pharmacology, Biochemistry and Behaviour 6: 343-347 (1977).

Alary, J.D.; Guay, P. and Brodeur, J.: Effect of phenobarbital pretreatment on the metabolism of DDT in
the rat and the bovine. Toxicology and Applied Pharmacology 18: 457-468 (1971).

American Academy of Pediatrics, Committee on Nutrition: Commentary on breast feeding and infant
formulas, including proposed standards for formulas. Pediatrics 57: 278 (1976).

American Academy of Pediatrics, Committee on Nutrition: Breast feeding: A commentary. Pediatrics 62:
591 (1978).

Amin-Zaki, L.; Elhassani, S.; Majeed, M.A.; Clarkson, T.W.; Doherty, R.A. and Greenwood, M.: Intra-
uterine methyl mercury poisoning in Iraq. Pediatrics 54: 587-595 (1974a).

Amin-Zaki, L.; Elhassani, S.; Majeed, M.A.; Clarkson, T.W.; Doherty, R.A. and Greenwood, M.R.:
Studies of infants postnatally exposed to methyl mercury. Journal of Pediatrics 85: 81-84 (1974b).

Amin-Zaki, L.; Elhassani, S.; Majeed, M.A.; Clarkson, T.W.; Doherty, R.A.; Greenwood, M.R. and Giovanoli-Jakubczak, T.: Perinatal methyl mercury poisoning in Iraq. American Journal of Diseases of Children 130: 1070-1076 (1976).

Ammon, H.V. and Phillips, S.F.: Inhibition of colonic water and electrolyte absorption by fatty acids in man. Gastroenterology 65: 744-749 (1973).

Ammon, H.V. and Phillips, S.F.: Inhibition of ileal water absorption by intraluminal fatty acids. Influence of chain length, hydroxylation, and conjugation of fatty acids. Journal of Clinical Investigation 53: 205-210 (1974).

Ammon, H.V.; Thomas, P.J. and Phillips, S.F.: Effects of oleic and ricinoleic acids on net jejunal water and electrolyte movement. Journal of Clinical Investigation 53: 374-379 (1974).

Ananth, J.: Side effects in the neonate from psychotropic agents excreted through breast-feeding. American Journal of Psychiatry 135: 801-805 (1978).

Anderson, P.O.: Drugs and breast feeding. Drug Intelligence and Clinical Pharmacy 11: 208-223 (1977).

Anderson, P. and Salter, F.: Propranolol therapy during pregnancy and lactation. American Journal of Cardiology 37: 325 (1976).

Applebaum, R.M.: The obstetrician's approach to the breasts and breast feeding. Journal of Reproductive Medicine 14: 98 (1975).

Aranda, J.V.; Sitar, D.S.; Parsons, W.D.; Loughnan, P.M. and Neims, A.H.: Pharmacokinetic aspects of theophylline in premature newborns. New England Journal of Medicine 295: 413-416 (1976).

Arena, J.M.: Drugs and breast feeding. Clinical Pediatrics 5: 472 (1966).

Atkinson, S.A.; Bryan, M.H. and Anderson, G.H.: Human milk: Difference in nitrogen concentration in milk from mothers of term and premature infants. Journal of Pediatrics 93: 67-69 (1978).

Avery, G.S.: Appendix A, Drug data information; in Avery (Ed): Drug Treatment, pp.888-896 (Adis Press, Sydney; Publishing Sciences Group, Acton, Mass.; Churchill-Livingstone, Edinburgh 1976a).

Avery, G.S.: Appendix E: Guide to drug dosage in renal failure; in Avery (Ed) Drug Treatment, pp.964-975 (Adis Press, Sydney; Publishing Sciences Group, Acton, Mass.; Churchill-Livingstone, Edinburgh 1976b).

Avner, S.E.: β-Adrenergic bronchodilators. Pediatric Clinics of North America 22: 129-139 (1975).

Ayd, F.J. (Ed): Excretion of psychotropic drugs in human breast milk. International Drug Therapy Newsletter, Vol. VIII: 33-40 (1973).

Bagnell, P.C. and Ellenberger, H.A.: Obstructive jaundice due to a chlorinated hydrocarbon in breast milk. Canadian Medical Association Journal 117: 1047-1048 (1977).

Bakir, F.; Damluji, S.F.; Amin-Zaki, L.; Murtadha, M.; Khalidi, A.; Al-Kawi, N.Y.; Tikriti, S.; Dhahir, H.I.; Clarkson, T.W.; Smith, J.C. and Doherty, R.A.: Methyl mercury poisoning in Iraq. Science 181: 230-241 (1973).

Bakken, A.F. and Seip, M.: Insecticides in human breast milk. Acta Paediatrica Scandinavica 65: 535-539 (1976).

Baldwin, W.F.: Clinical study of senna administration to nursing mothers: Assessment of effects on infant bowel habits. Canadian Medical Association Journal 89: 566-568 (1963).

Bambel, C.E. and Hunter, R.E.: Effect of dicoumarol on the nursing infant. American Journal of Obstetrics and Gynecology 59: 1153-1159 (1950).

Banerjee, N.C.; Miller, G.E. and Stowe, C.M.: Excretion of aminopyrine and its metabolites into cows milk. Toxicology and Applied Pharmacology 10: 604-612 (1967).

Barness, L.A.: Breast milk for all. New England Journal of Medicine 297(17): 939-941 (1977).

Barrie, H.; Martin, E. and Ansell, C.: Milks for babies. Lancet 2: 1330 (1975).

Bartig, D. and Cohon, M.: Excretion of drugs in human milk. Hospital Formulary Management 4: 26-27 (1969).

Baty, J.D.; Breckenridge, A.; Lewis, P.J.; Orme, M.; Serlin, M.J. and Sibeon, R.G.: May mothers taking warfarin breast feed their infants? British Journal of Clinical Pharmacology 3: 969 (1976).

Bauer, J.H.; Pape, B.; Zajicek, J. and Groshong, T.: Propranolol in human plasma and breast milk. American Journal of Cardiology 43: 860-862 (1979).

Beer, A.E. and Billingham, R.E.: Immunologic benefits and hazards of milk in maternal perinatal relationship. Annals of Internal Medicine 83: 865-871 (1975).

Bell, K. and McKenzie, H.A.: β-Lactoglobulins. Nature 204: 1275 (1964).

Berlin, C.M. Jr.; Pascuzzi, M.J. and Yaffe, S.J.: Excretion of salicylate in human milk (Abst). Clinical Pharmacology and Therapeutics 27: 245 (1980).

Binder, H.J.: Pharmacology of laxatives. Annual Review of Pharmacology and Toxicology 17: 355-367 (1977).

Binder, R.G.; Applewhite, T.H.; Kohler, G.C. and Goldblatt, L.A.: Chromatographic analysis of seed oils. Fatty acid composition of castor oil. Journal of the American Oil Chemists Society 39: 513-517 (1962).

Binkiewicz, A.; Robinson, M.J. and Senior, B.: Pseudo-Cushing syndrome caused by alcohol in breast milk. Journal of Pediatrics 93: 965 (1978).

Bisdom, C.J.W.: Alcohol and nicotine poisoning in nurslings. Maandschrift voor Kindergeneeskunde 6: 332 (1937).

Blacker, K.H.; Weinstein, B.J. and Ellman, G.L.: Mother's milk and chlorpromazine. American Journal of Psychiatry 119: 178-179 (1962).

Blaikley, J.B.; Clarke, S.; MacKeith, R. and Ogden, K.M.: Breast-feeding: Factors affecting success. Journal of Obstetrics and Gynaecology of the British Empire 60: 657-669 (1953).

Blau, S.P.: Metabolism of gold during lactation. Arthritis and Rheumatism 16: 777-778 (1973).

Blinick, G.; Inturrisi, C.E.; Jerez, E. and Wallach, R.C.: Methadone assays in pregnant women and progeny. American Journal of Obstetrics and Gynecology 121: 617-621 (1975).

Bond, C.A. and Woodham, D.W.: The cumulation and disappearance of mirex residues. II. In milk and tissues of cows fed two concentrations of the insecticide in their diet. Bulletin of Environmental Contamination and Toxicology 14: 25-31 (1975).

Bostock, J.: Evolutionary approaches to infant care. Lancet 1: 1033-1035 (1962).

Brandt, R.: Passage of diazepam and desmethyldiazepam into breast milk. Arzneimittel-Forschung 26: 454-457 (1976).

Breimer, D.D. and Baars, A.J.: Pharmacokinetics and metabolism of anthraquinone laxatives. Pharmacology 14(Suppl. 1): 30-47 (1976).

Brew, K.: Secretion of α-lactalbumin into milk and its relevance to the organization and control of lactose synthetase. Nature 222: 671-672 (1969).

Bright-Asare, P. and Binder, H.J.: Stimulation of colonic secretion of water and electrolytes by hydroxy fatty acids. Gastroenterology 64: 81-88 (1973).

Brodbeck, U. and Ebner, K.E.: Resolution of a soluble lactose syntherase into two protein components and solublimation of microsomal lactose syntherase. Journal of Biological Chemistry 241: 762-764 (1966).

Brodbeck, U.; Denton, W.L.; Tanahashi, N. and Ebner, K.E.: The isolation and identification of the β protein of lactose as α-lactalbumin. Journal of Biological Chemistry 242: 1391-1397 (1967).

Brodie, B.B.: Physico-chemical factors in drug absorption; in Absorption and Distribution of Drugs (Livingstone, Edinburgh-London 1964).

Brodie, B.B. and Hogben, C.A.M.: Some physico-chemical factors in drug action. Journal of Pharmacy and Pharmacology 9: 345-380 (1957).

Brown, D.R.: Neonatal lead exposure in the rat: Decreased learning as a function of age and blood level concentrations. Toxicology and Applied Pharmacology 32: 628-637 (1975).

Brown, R.D. and Manno, J.E.: ESTRIP, a BASIC Computer Program for obtaining initial polyexponential parameter estimates. Journal of Pharmaceutical Sciences 67(12): 1687-1691 (1978).

Brown-Grant, K.: The iodide concentrating mechanism of the mammary gland. Journal of Physiology (London) 135: 644-654 (1957).

Buchanan, R.A.; Eaton, C.J.; Koeff, S.T. and Kinkel, A.W.: The breast milk excretion of mefenamic acid. Current Therapeutic Research 10: 592-596 (1968).

Buchanan, R.A.; Eaton, C.J.; Koeff, S.T. and Kinkel, A.W.: The breast milk excretion of flufenamic acid. Current Therapeutic Research 11: 533-538 (1969).

Bucher, T. and Redetzki, H.: Eine spezifische-photometrische Restimmung von Athylalkohol auf fermentativem Wege. Klinische Wochenschrift 29: 615 (1951).

Buckalew, L.W.: Effect of maternal alcohol consumption during nursing on offspring activity. Research Communications in Psychology, Psychiatry, and Behaviour 3: 353-358 (1978).

Burt, G.S.: Use of behavioural techniques in the assessment of environmental contaminants; in Weiss and Laties (Eds) Behavioral Toxicology, pp.241-262 (Plenum Press, New York, 1975).

Byck, R.: Drugs and the treatment of psychiatric disorder; in Goodman and Gilman (Eds) The Pharmacological Basis of Therapeutics, pp.152-200 (Macmillan Publishing Company, New York 1975).

Castell, D.O. and Levine, S.M.: Lower esophageal sphincter response to gastric neutralization. A new mechanism for treatment of heartburn with antacids. Annals of Internal Medicine 74: 223-227 (1971).

Catz, C.S. and Giacoia, G.P.: Drugs and breast milk. Pediatric Clinics of North America 19: 151-166 (1972).

Chan, V.; Tse, T.F. and Wong, V.: Transfer of digoxin across the placenta and into breast milk. British Journal of Obstetrics and Gynaecology (London) 85: 605-609 (1978).

Chao, F-C.; Green, D.E.; Forrest, I.S.; Kaplan, J.N.; Winship-Ball, A. and Brande, M.: The passage of ^{14}C-D-9-tetrahydrocannabinol into the milk of lactating squirrel monkeys. Research Communications in Chemical Pathology and Pharmacology 15: 303-317 (1976).

Clayman, C.B.: Evaluation of cimetidine (Tagamet). An antagonist of hydrochloric acid secretion. Journal of the American Medical Association 238: 1289-1290 (1977).

Clyde, D.F. and Shute, G.T.: Transfer of pyrimethamine in human milk. Journal of Tropical Medicine and Hygiene, December: 277-287 (1956).

Cobo, E.: Effect of different doses of ethanol on the milk-ejecting reflex in lactating women. American Journal of Obstetrics and Gynecology 115: 817-819 (1973).

Cobrinik, R.W.; Hood, R.T. and Chusid, E.: The effect of maternal narcotic addiction on the newborn infant. Pediatrics 24: 288-304 (1959).

Cole, A.P. and Hailey, D.M.: Diazepam and active metabolite in breast milk and their transfer to the neonate. Archives of Disease in Childhood (London) 50: 741-742 (1975).

Conney, A.H.: Pharmacological implications of microsomal enzyme induction. Pharmacological Reviews 19: 317-366 (1967).

Coradello, H.: The excretion of antiepileptic drugs in breast milk. Wiener Klinische Wochenschrift 85: 695-697 (1973).

Cote, C.J.; Kenepp, N.B.; Reed, S.B. and Strobel, G.E.: Trace concentrations of halothane in human breast milk. British Journal of Anaesthesia 48: 541-543 (1976).

Cueto, C. Jr. and Hayes, W.J. Jr.: Effect of phenobarbital on the metabolism of dieldrin. Toxicology and Applied Pharmacology 7: 481 (1965).

Cunningham, A.S.: Morbidity in breast-fed and artificially fed infants. Journal of Pediatrics 90: 726 (1977).

Curley, A. and Kimbrough, R.: Chlorinated hydrocarbon insecticides in plasma and milk of pregnant and lactating women. Archives of Environmental Health 18: 156-164 (1969).

Curry, S.H.; Riddall, D.; Gordon, J.S.; Simpson, P.; Binns, T.B.; Rondel, R.K. and McMartin, C.: Disposition of glutethimide in man. Clinical Pharmacology and Therapeutics 12: 849-857 (1971).

Cuthbertson, W.F.: Essential fatty acid requirements in infancy. American Journal of Clinical Nutrition 29: 559 (1976).

Daly, J.C.; Goodyear, S.; Paperiello, C.J. and Matuszek, J.M.: Iodine-129 levels in milk and water near a nuclear fuel reprocessing plant. Health Physics 26: 333-342 (1974).

Darlington, R.C.: Laxative products; in Handbook of Nonprescription Drugs, pp.36-53 (American Pharmaceutical Association, Washington, D.C. 1977).

Davson, H. and Danielli, J.F.: The Permeability of Natural Membranes, 2nd Ed. (Cambridge University Press, London 1943).

Deb, A.K. and Cama, H.R.: Studies in human lactation. British Journal of Nutrition 16: 65 (1962).

Devlin, R.G. and Fleiss, P.M.: Selective resistance to the passage of captopril into human milk (Abst). Clinical Pharmacology and Therapeutics 27: 250 (1980).

Dews, P.B. and Morse, W.H.: Behavioral pharmacology. Annual Review of Pharmacology 1: 145-174 (1961).

Dieterle, W.; Wagner, J. and Faigle, J.W.: Binding of chlorthalidone (Hygroton) to blood components in man. Journal of Clinical Pharmacology 10: 37-42 (1976).

Dillon, H.K.; Wilson, D.J. and Schaffner, W.: Lead concentrations in human milk. American Journal of Diseases of Children 128: 491-492 (1974).

Dujovne, C.A. and Shoeman, D.W.: Toxicity of a hepatotoxic laxative preparation in tissue culture and excretion in bile in man. Clinical Pharmacology and Therapeutics 13: 602-608 (1972).

Durham, W.F.: Body burdens of pesticides in man. Annals of the New York Academy of Science 160: 183-195 (1969).

Dyment, P.G.; Hebertson, L.M.; Decker, W.J.; Gomes, E.D. and Wiseman, J.S.: Relationship between levels of chlorinated hydrocarbon insecticides in human milk and serum. Bulletin of Environmental Contamination and Toxicology 6: 449-452 (1971a).

Dyment, P.G.; Hebertson, L.M.; Gomes, E.D.; Wiseman, J.S. and Hornabrook, R.W.: Absence of polychlorinated biphenyls in human milk and serum from Texas and human milk from New Guinea. Bulletin of Environmental Contamination and Toxicology 6: 532-534 (1971b).

Eckert, C.D.; Sloan, M.V.; Duncan, J.R. and Hurley, L.S.: Zinc binding: a difference between human and bovine milk. Science 195: 789-790 (1977).

Eckstein, H.B. and Jack, B.: Breast feeding and anticoagulant therapy. Lancet 1: 672-673 (1970).

Edozien, J.C.; Khan, R.M.A. and Washien, C.I.: Protein deficiency in man: Results of a Nigerian village study. Journal of Nutrition 106: 312 (1976).

Emery, W.B.; Canolty, N.L.; Aitchison, J.M. and Dunkley, W.L.: Influence of sampling on fatty acid composition of human milk. American Journal of Clinical Nutrition 31: 1127-1130 (1978).

Engel, J. and Lundborg, P.: Regional changes in monoamine levels and in the rate of tyrosine and tryptophan hydroxylation in 4 week old offspring of nursing mothers treated with the neuroleptic drug penfluridol. Naunyn-Schmiedeberg's Archives of Pharmacology 282: 327-334 (1974).

Erkkola, R. and Kanto, J.: Diazepam and breast-feeding. Lancet 1: 1235-1236 (1972).

Eschenhof, V.E. and Rieder, J.: Untersuchungen uber das schicksal des antidepressivums amitriptylin im organismus der ratte und des menschen. Arzneimittel Forschung 19: 957-966 (1969).

Evans, P.R. and MacKeith, R.C.: Infant Feeding and Feeding Difficulties, 3rd Ed., p.71 (Churchill-Livingstone, London 1958).

Fahim, M.S. and King, T.M.: Effect of phenobarbital on lactation and the nursing neonate. American Journal of Obstetrics and Gynecology 101: 1103-1108 (1968).

Fantus, B. and Dyniewicz, J.W.: Phenolphthalein administration to nursing women. American Journal of Digestive Diseases 3: 184-185 (1936).

Federal Drug Administration Panel on OTC Laxatives, Antidiarrheals, Antiemetics and Emetic Drugs. Federal Register 40: 12924-12933 (1975).

Fehily, L.: Human milk intoxication due to B_1 avitaminosis. British Medical Journal 2: 590-592 (1944).

Ferguson, B.B.; Wilson, D.J. and Schaffner, W.: Determination of nicotine concentrations in human milk. American Journal of Diseases of Children 130: 837-839 (1976).

Findlay, J.W.A.; DeAngelis, R.L.; Kearney, M.F.; Welch, R.M. and Findlay, J.M.: Analgesic drugs in breast milk and plasma (Abst). World Conference on Clinical Pharamcology, London (1980).

Fingl, E.: Laxatives and cathartics; in Goodman and Gilman (Eds) The Pharmacological Basis of Therapeutics, pp.976-986 (Macmillan Publishing Company, New York 1975).

Finley, J.P., Waxman, M.B.; Wong, P.Y. and Lickrish, G.M.: Digoxin excretion in human milk. Journal of Pediatrics 94: 339-340 (1979).

Flanagan, T.L.; Lin, T.H.; Novick, W.J.; Rondish, I.M.; Bocher, C.A. and Van Loon, E.J.: Spectrophotometric method for the determination of chlorpromazine and chlorpromazine sulphoxide in biological fluids. Journal of Medicinal and Pharmaceutical Chemistry 1: 263-273 (1959).

Fomon, S.J.: Infant Nutrition, 2nd Ed. (W.B. Saunders Company, Philadelphia 1974).

Fouts, J.R. and Hart, L.G.: Hepatic drug metabolism in the perinatal period. Annals of the New York Academy of Sciences 123: 245-251 (1965).

Friebel, H. and Walkowiak, L.: The detection of purgative drugs containing anthraquinone in human milk. Archives fur Gynakologie 179: 123-135 (1951).

Fries, G.F.; Marrow, G.S., Jr; Lester, J.W. and Gordon, C.H.: Effect of microsomal enzyme inducing drugs on DDT and dieldrin elimination from cows. Journal of Dairy Science 54: 364-368 (1971).

Frontali, G.: Sull' importanze clinica des passaglo d'alcohol attraverso la glandula mammaria. Revista di Clinica Pediatrica 13: 693 (1915).

Fujita, M. and Takabutake, E.: Mercury levels in human maternal and neonatal blood, hair and milk. Bulletin of Environmental Contamination and Toxicology 18: 205-209 (1977).

Gadacz, T.R.; Gaginella, T.S. and Phillips, S.F.: Inhibition of water absorption by ricinoleic acid. Evidence against hormonal mediation of the effect. American Journal of Digestive Diseases 21: 859-862 (1976).

Gaginella, T.S. and Bass, P.: Laxatives: An update on mechanisms of action. Life Sciences 23: 1001-1010 (1978).

Gaginella, T.S. and Phillips, S.F.: Ricinoleic acid (castor oil) alters intestinal surface structure. Mayo Clinic Proceedings 51: 6-12 (1976).

Gaginella, T.S.; Stewart, J.J.; Gullikson, G.W.; Olsen, W.A. and Bass, P.: Inhibition of small intestinal mucosal and smooth muscle cell function by ricinoleic acid and other surfactants. Life Sciences 16: 1595-1606 (1975a).

Gaginella, T.S.; Stewart, J.J.; Olsen, W.A. and Bass, P: Actions of ricinoleic acid and structurally related fatty acids on the gastrointestinal tract. II. Effects on water and electrolyte absorption in vitro. Journal of Pharmacology and Experimental Therapeutics 195: 355-361 (1975b).

Garcia, J.D.; Yang, M.G.; Belo, P.S. and Wang, J.H.C.: Carbon-mercury bond breakage in milk, cerebrum, liver and kidney of rats fed methyl mercury chloride. Proceedings of the Society for Experimental Biology and Medicine 146: 190-193 (1974).

Gauron, E.F. and Rowley, V.N.: Effects on offspring behavior of parental early drug experience and cross-fostering. Psychopharmacologia 30: 269-274 (1973).

Glenn, J.C. and Hansard, S.C.: Mammary iron transfer in lactating ewes. Journal of Animal Science 23: 905 (1964).

Godding, E.W.: Therapeutics of laxative agents with special reference to the anthraquinones. Pharmacology 14 (Suppl. 1): 78-101 (1976).

Gopalan, C.: Studies on lactation in poor Indian communities. Journal of Tropical Pediatrics 4: 87 (1958).

Gopalan C. and Belavady, B.: Nutrition and Lactation. Federation Proceedings 20 (1), Part 3 (1961).

Gostof, Homolka and Zelenka: Les substances derivees du tromexane dans le lait maternel et leurs actions paradoxales sur la prothrombine. Schweizerische Medizinische Wochenschrift 30: 764-765 (1952).

Govind-Rao, M.K.; Risser, N. and Perkins, E.G.: The incorporation of ricinoleic acid into rat lymph lipids. Proceedings of the Society for Experimental Biology and Medicine 131: 1369-1372 (1969).

Greene, H.J.; Burkhart, B. and Hobby, D.G.L.: Excretion of penicillin in human milk following parturition. American Journal of Obstetrics and Gynecology 51: 732-733 (1946).

Greenleaf, J.O. and Leonard, H.S.D.: Laxatives in the treatment of constipation in pregnant and breast-feeding mothers. Practitioner 210: 259-263 (1973).

Gruner, O.: Der Gerichtsmedizinische Alkoholnachwies, 2nd Ed., p.44 (Carl Heymanns Verlag KG, Cologne 1967).

Gustafson, P.E. and Miller, J.E.: The significance of ^{137}Cs in man and his diet. Health Physics 16: 167-183 (1969).

Guthrie, H.A.; Picciano, M.F. and Sheehe, D.: Fatty acid patterns of human milk. Journal of Pediatrics 90: 39-41 (1977).

Gyrd-Hansen, af N. and Rasmussen, F.: Renal og mammaer ekskretion af lincomycin hos koer. Scandinavian Journal of Veterinary Science 19: 11-16 (1967).

Hagyard, S.B.; Brown, W.H.; Stull, J.W.; Whiting, F.M. and Kemberling, S.R.: DDT and DDE content of human milk in Arizona. Bulletin of Environmental Contamination and Toxicology 9: 169-172 (1973).

Hall, B.: Changing composition of human milk and early development of appetite control. Lancet 1: 779-781 (April 5, 1975).

Hambraeus, L.: Proprietary milk versus human breast milk in infant feeding. A critical appraisal from the nutritional point of view. Pediatric Clinics of North America 24 (1): 17-36 (1977).

Hambraeus, L.; Forsum, E. and Lonnerdal, B.: Nutritional aspects of breast milk versus cow's milk formula; in McFarlane, Hambraeus and Hanson (Eds) Food and Immunology. Symposia of the Swedish Nutrition Foundation XIII. (Almqvist and Wiksell, Stockholm 1976).

Hanwell, A. and Linzell, J.L.: Elevation of the cardiac output in the rat by prolactin and growth hormone. Journal of Endocrinology 53: 57-58 (1972).

Hanwell, A. and Linzell, J.L.: The effects of engorgement with milk and of suckling on mammary blood flow in the rat. Journal of Physiology 233: 111-125 (1973).

Hartmann, P.E. and Kulski, J.K.: Changes in the composition of the mammary secretion of women after abrupt termination of breast feeding. Journal of Physiology 275: 1-11 (1978).

Havelka, J.; Hejzlar, M.; Popov, V.; Viktorinova, D. and Prochazka, J.: Excretion of chloramphenicol in human milk. Chemotherapy 13: 204-211 (1968).

Hawthorne, J.C.; Ford, J.H.; Loftis, C.D. and Markin, G.P.: Mirex in milk from southeastern United States. Bulletin of Environmental Contamination and Toxicology 11: 238-240 (1974).

Hayes, W.J.: Review of the metabolism of chlorinated hydrocarbon insecticides especially in mammals. Annual Review of Pharmacology 5: 27-52 (1965).

Hayes, W.J.: Dosage relationships associated with DDT in milk. Toxicology and Applied Pharmacology 38: 19-28 (1976).

Healy, M.: Suppressing lactation with oral diuretics. Lancet 1: 1353-1354 (1961).

Hebb, C.O. and Linzell, J.L.: Some conditions affecting the blood flow through the perfused mammary gland, with special reference to the action of adrenaline. Quarterly Journal of Experimental Physiology 36: 159-175 (1951).

Herting, D.C. and Drury, E.E.: Thin-layer chromatography with precoated alumina sheets II. Application to tocopherols. Journal of Chromatography 30: 502-505 (1967).

Hervada, A.R.; Feit, E. and Sagraves, R.: Drugs in breast milk. Perinatal Care 2: 19-25 (1978).

Hoh, T.K.: Severe hypoprothrombinaemic bleeding in the breast fed young infants. Singapore Medical Journal 10: 43-49 (1969).

Hollman, K.H.: Cytology and fine structure of the mammary gland; in Larson and Smith (Eds) Lactation: A Comprehensive Treatise. I. The Mammary Gland/Development and Maintenance (Academic Press, New York/London 1974).

Hornabrook, R.W.; Dyment, P.G.; Gomes, E.D. and Wiseman, J.S.: DDT residues in human milk from New Guinea natives. Medical Journal of Australia 1: 1297-1300 (1972).

Horning, M.G.; Nowlin, J.; Hickert, P.; Stilwell, W.G. and Hill, R.M.: Identification of drugs and drug metabolites in breast milk by gas chromatography - mass spectrometry; M. Galli (Ed). Dietary Lipids and Postnatal Development, pp.257-269 (Raven Press, New York 1973).

Horning, M.G.; Stillwell, W.G.; Nowlin, J.; Lertratanangkoon, K.; Stillwell, R.N. and Hill, R.M.: Identification and quantification of drugs and drug metabolites in human breast milk using GC-MS-COM methods. Modern Problems in Paediatrics 15: 73-79 (1975).

Hytten, F.E.: Clinical and chemical studies in human lactation. British Medical Journal 1: 175-182 (1954).

Hytten, F.E. and Leitch, I.: The Physiology of Human Pregnancy, 2nd Ed. (Blackworld Scientific Publications, Oxford 1971).

Illingworth, R.S.: Abnormal substances excreted in human milk. Practitioner 171: 533-538 (1953).

Illingworth, R.S. and Finch, E.: Ethyl bisconmacetate (Tromexan) in human milk. Journal of Obstetrics and Gynaecology of the British Empire 66: 487-488 (1959).

Innes, I.R. and Nickerson, M.: Atropine, scopolamine, and related antimuscarinic drugs: in Goodman and Gilman (Eds) The Pharmacological Basis of Therapeutics, pp.514-532 (Macmillan Publishing Company, New York 1975).

Insull, W.; Hirsch, J.; James, T. and Ahrens, E.H.: The fatty acids of human milk. II. Alterations produced by manipulation of caloric balance and exchange of dietary fats. Journal of Clinical Investigation 38: 443 (1959).

Irvin, R.R.: Caffeine in the breast milk of coffee and tea drinkers. Medical Journal and Record 124: 37-38 (1926).

Jack, D.; Harris, D.M. and Middleton, E., Jr: Adrenergic agents; in Middleton, Reed and Ellis (Eds) Allergy Principles and Practice, pp.404-433 (Mosby, St. Louis 1978).

Jacobs, M.H.: Some aspects of cell permeability to weak electrolytes. Cold Spring Harbor Symposia on Quantitative Biology 8: 30 (1940).

Jakubovic, A.; Tait, R.M. and McGeer, P.L.: Excretion of THC and its metabolites in ewes' milk. Toxicology and Applied Pharmacology 28: 38-43 (1974).

Jan, J.; Komar, M. and Milohnoja, M.: Excretion of some pure PCB isomers in milk of cows. Bulletin of Environmental Contamination and Toxicology 13: 313-315 (1975).

Jelliffe, D.B.: The secotrant — a possible new category in early childhood. Journal of Pediatrics 74: 808-810 (1969).

Jelliffe, D.B. and Jelliffe, E.F.P.: The effects of starvation on the function of the family and of society; in Blix and Vahlqvist (Eds) Nutrition and Relief Operations in Times of Disaster. (Almqvist and Wilsells, Uppsala 1971).

Jelliffe, D.B. and Jelliffe, E.F.P.: Alleged inadequacies of human milk: Common misapprehensions and errors. Clinical Pediatrics 16: 1140-1144 (1977a).

Jelliffe, D.B. and Jelliffe, E.F.P.: Current concepts on nutrition. New England Journal of Medicine 297: 912-915 (1977b).

Jelliffe, D.B. and Jelliffe, E.F.P.: Human Milk in the Modern World (Oxford University Press, London 1977c).

Jelliffe, D.B. and Jelliffe, E.F.P.: The volume and composition of human milk in poorly nourished communities — a review. American Journal of Clinical Nutrition 31: 492-515 (1978).

Johannson, I.; Korkman, N. and Nelson, N.J.: Studies on udder evacuation in dairy cows. I. The rise in fat percentage during milking. Acta Agriculturae Scandinavica 2: 43-81 (1952).

Johns, D.G.; Rutherford, L.D.; Keighton, P.C. and Vogel, C.L.: Secretion of methotrexate into human milk. American Journal of Obstetrics and Gynecology 112: 978-980 (1972).

Jusko, W.J. and Pliszezuk, A.: Analysis of theophylline in biological fluids by HPLC: in Dupont Liquid Chromatography Applications Report (DuPont Instruments, Wilmington, Delaware 1975).

Juul, S.: Fenemalforgittning via modermaelken? Uneskrift for Laeger 131: 2257-2258 (1976).

Kadlec, G.J.; Ha, L.T.; Jarboe, C.H.; Richards, D.R. and Karibo, J.M.: Theophylline half-life in infants and young children. Annals of Allergy 40: 303-310 (1978).

Kahn, H.L. and Kerber, J.D.: Sampling improvements in atomic absorption spectroscopy. Journal of the American Oil Chemists Society 48: 434-437 (1971).

Kaneko, S.; Sato, T. and Suzuki, K.: The levels of anticonvulsants in breast milk. British Journal of Clinical Pharmacology 7: 624-629 (1979).

Karpow, S.; Gotz, V. and Lauper, R.D.: Cimetidine. Journal of the American Medical Association 239: 402 (1978).

Kampman, J.P.; Johansen, K.; Hanson, J.M. and Helweg, J.: Propylthiouracil in human milk. The Lancet: 736-737 (1980).

Katz, F. and Duncan, B.R.: Entry of prednisone into human milk. Archives of Disease in Childhood 50: 894-896 (1975a).

Katz, F. and Duncan, B.R.: Entry of prednisone into human milk. New England Journal of Medicine 293: 1154 (1975b).

Keenan, T.W.; Morre, D.J. and Cheetham, R.D.: Lactose synthesis by a Golgi apparatus fraction from rat mammary gland. Nature 228: 1105-1106 (1970).

Kesaniemi, Y.A.: Ethanol and acetaldehyde in the milk and peripheral blood of lactating women after ethanol administration. Journal of Obstetrics and Gynaecology of the British Commonwealth 81: 84-86 (1974).

Khazen, K.; Mishkinsky, J.; Ben-David, M. and Sulmon, F.G.: Lactogenic effect of phenothiazine-like drugs. Archives Internationales de Pharmacodynamie et de Therapie 174: 428-441 (1968).

Klaus, M.H. and Kennell, J.H.: Mother-infant bonding: The impact of early separation or loss on family development (Mosby, St. Louis 1976).

Klaus, M.H.; Kennell, J.H.; Plumb, N. and Zuehlke, S.: Human maternal behaviour at the first contact with her young. Pediatrics 46: 187-192 (1970).

Klausner, H.A. and Dingell, J.V.: The metabolism and excretion of Δ⁹-tetrahydrocannabinol in the rat. Life Sciences 10: 49-59 (1971).

Klemmer, H.W.; Budy, A.M.; Takahashi, W. and Haley, T.J.: Human tissue distribution of cyclodiene pesticides — Hawaii 1964-1973. Clinical Toxicology 11: 71-82 (1977).

Knowles, J.A.: Excretion of drugs in milk — A review. Journal of Pediatrics 66: 1068-1082 (1965).

Knowles, J.A.: Drugs in milk. Ross Timesaver Pediatric Currents 21: 28-32 (1972).

Knowles, J.A.: Effects on the infant of drug therapy in nursing mothers. Drug Therapy 3: 57-65 (1973).

Knowles, J.A.: Breast milk: A source of more than nutrition for the neonate. Clinical Toxicology 7: 69-82 (1974).

Knutsson, P.G.: Exchange of sodium, potassium, chloride, and phosphate ions across the mammary epithelium in the goat. Annual Report Agricultural College of Sweden 30: 477-506 (1964).

Knutsson, P.G. and Sperber, I.: Exchange of ions across mammary epithelium and the formation of milk; in Symposium on the use of radioisotopes in animal nutrition and physiology (SM-53/20, Prague 1964).

Kojima, K. and Araki, T.: Recent status of organochlorine pesticide residues in foods in Japan. Environmental Quality and Safety 4: 74-79 (1975).

Kolodny, R.C.; Jacobs, L.S. and Daughaday, W.H.: Mammary stimulation causes prolactin secretion in non-lactating women. Nature 238: 284-285 (1972).

Kon, S.K. and Mawson, E.H.: Milk and mammary gland and its secretion. Medical Research Council Special Report Series 269 (1950).

Koup, J.R.: Principles of therapeutics; in Middleton, Reed and Ellis (Eds) Allergy, Principles and Practice, pp.388-403 (Mosby, St. Louis 1978).

Kreek, M.J.; Schecter, A.; Gutjahr, C.L.; Bowen, D.; Field, F.; Pueenan, J. and Merkatz, I.: Analyses of methadone and other drugs in maternal and neonatal fluids: Use in evaluation of symptoms in a neonate of mother maintained on methadone. American Journal of Drug and Alcohol Abuse 1: 409-419 (1974).

Kroger, M.: Insecticide residues in human milk. Journal of Pediatrics 80: 401-405 (1972).

Kroger, M.: General environmental contaminants occurring in milk; in Larson and Smith (Eds) Lactation: A Comprehensive Treatise, Vol. III: Nutrition and Biochemistry of Milk/Maintenance (Academic

Press, New York 1974).

Krzeminski, L.F.; Cox, B.L.; Perrel, P.N. and Schlitz, R.A.: Determination of methylprednisolone (Medrol) residues in milk by high pressure liquid chromatography. Journal of Agricultural and Food Chemistry 20: 970-972 (1972).

Kulski, J.K.; Hartmann, P.E.; Martin, J.D. and Smith, M.: Effects of bromocriptine mesylate on the composition of the mammary secretion in non-breast feeding women. Obstetrics and Gynecology 52: 38-42 (1978).

Kwit, N.T. and Hatcher, R.A.: Excretion of drugs in milk. American Journal of Diseases of Children 49: 900-904 (1935).

Ladinskaya, L.A.; Parfenov, Y.D.; Popov, D.K. and Fedorova, A.V.: ^{210}Pb and ^{210}Po content in air, water, foodstuffs and the human body. Archives of Environmental Health 27: 254-258 (1973).

Levin, R.J.; Moore, R.M.; McLaren, G.D.; Barthel, W.F. and Landrigan, P.J.: Occupational lead poisoning, animal deaths, and environmental contamination at a scrap smelter. American Journal of Public Health 66: 548-552 (1976).

Levitan, A.A. and Manion, J.C.: Propranolol therapy during pregnancy and lactation. American Journal of Cardiology 32: 247 (1973).

Levy, M.; Granit, L. and Laufer, N.: Excretion of drugs in human milk. New England Journal of Medicine 294: 789 (1977).

Lindblad, B.S.; Ljungquist, M.; Meldin, G. and Rahimtoola, R.J.: Food and immunology: The composition and yield of human milk in developing countries. Proceedings of the Swedish Nutrition Symposium (1976).

Lindblad, B.S. and Rahimtoola, R.J.: A pilot study of the quality of human milk in a lower socioeconomic group in Karachi, Pakistan. Acta Paediatrica Scandinavica 63: 125 (1974).

Linzell, J.L.: Vasomotor nerve fibers to mammary glands of the cat and dog. Quarterly Journal of Experimental Physiology 35: 259-319 (1950).

Linzell, J.L.: The flow and composition of mammary gland lymph. Journal of Physiology (London) 153: 510-521 (1960).

Linzell, J.L.: The effect of the very frequent milking and of oxytocin on the yield and composition of milk in fed and fasted goats. Journal of Physiology (London) 190: 333-346 (1967).

Linzell, J.L.: Mammary blood flow and methods of identifying and measuring precursors of milk; in Larson and Smith (Eds) Lactation, Vol. 1, pp.143-225 (Academic Press, New York 1974).

Linzell, J.L. and Peaker, M.: Intracellular concentrations of sodium, potassium and chloride in the lactating mammary gland and their relation to the secretory mechanism. Journal of Physiology (London) 216: 683-700 (1971a).

Linzell, J.L. and Peaker, M.: The permeability of mammary ducts. Journal of Physiology (London) 216: 701-716 (1971b).

Linzell, J.L. and Peaker, M.: Mechanism of milk secretion. Physiological Reviews 51: 564-597 (1971c).

Lipman, A.G.: Antimicrobial agents in breast milk. Modern Medicine, March 15: 89-90 (1977).

Livingston, S.: Treatment of epilepsy with diphenylhydantoin sodium. Postgraduate Medicine 201: 584-590 (1956).

Lombeck, I.; Kasperek, K.; Bonnermann, B.; Feinendegan, L.E. and Bremer, H.J.: Selenium content of human milk, cow's milk and cow's milk infant formulas. European Journal of Pediatrics 129: 139-145 (1978).

Lonnerdal, B.; Forsum, E. and Hambraeus, L.: The protein content of human milk. Proceedings of the Tenth International Congress of Nutrition, Kyoto, Japan: Victroy-sha Press, p.698 (1976a).

Lonnerdal, B.; Forsum, E. and Hambraeus, L.: A longitudinal study of the protein, nitrogen, and lactose contents of human milk from Swedish well-nourished mothers. The American Journal of Clinical Nutrition 29: 1127-1133 (1976b).

Lonnerdal, B.; Forsum, E. and Hambraeus, L.: A longitudinal study of the protein content of human milk from well-nourished Swedish mothers. Nutrition and Metabolism 21 (Suppl. 1): 106-109 (1977).

Loughnan, P.M.: Digoxin in human breast milk. Journal of Pediatrics 92: 1019-1020 (1978).

Lucas, A.; Gibbs, J.A.H.; Lyster, R.L.J. and Baum, J.D.: Creamatocrit: simple clinical technique for estimating fat concentration and energy value of human milk. British Medical Journal 1: 1018-1020 (1978).

Lundborg, P.: Abnormal ontogeny in young rabbits after chronic administration of haloperidol to the nursing mothers. Brain Research 44: 684-687 (1972).

Luquet, F.M.; Goursaud, J. and Casalis, J.: La pollution des laits humains francais par les residues d'insecticides organochlores. Pathologie Biologie 23: 45-49 (1975).

Luquet, F.M.; Goursaud, J. and Gaudier, B.: Etude de la pollution des laits humains par les residues de pesticides. Pathologie Biologie 20: 137-143 (1972).

Lynch, M.A.: Ill-health and child abuse. Lancet 2: 317-319 (1975).

McClanahan, B.J.; McClellan, R.D.; McDenny, J.R. and Bustard, L.K.: Symposium on radioisotopes in animals, nutrition and physiology. International Atomic Energy Agency Technical Report Series, Vienna 173: 88 (1965).

McKenzie, S.A.; Selley, J.A. and Agnew, J.E.: Secretion of prednisolone into breast milk. Archives of Disease in Childhood 50: 894-896 (1975).

Mackay, A.V.P.; Loose, R. and Glen, A.I.M.: Labor and lithium. British Medical Journal 1: 878 (1976).

Malven, P.V. and McMurtry, J.P.: Measurement of prolactin in milk by radioimmunoassay. Journal of Dairy Science 57: 411-415 (1974).

Manes, J.D.; Fluckiger, H.B. and Schneider, D.L.: Chromatographic analysis of Vitamin K_1; Application to infant formula products. Journal of Agriculture and Food Chemistry 20: 1130-1132 (1972).

Maricq, L. and Molle, L: Recherches sur la determination de l'alcoolemie par chromatographie gazeuse. Bulletin de L'Academie Royale de Medecine de Belgique 24: 199 (1959).

Masuda, Y.; Kagawa, R. and Kuratsune, M.: Comparison of polychlorinated biphenyls in Yusho patients and ordinary persons. Bulletin of Environmental Contamination and Toxicology 11: 213-216 (1974).

Mayo, C.C. and Schlicke, C.P.: Appearance of a barbiturate in human milk. Proceedings of the Staff Meetings of the Mayo Clinic 17: 87-88 (1942).

Mee, J.M.L.: Rapid determination of β-hydroxybutyric acid in blood and milk by gas chromatography. Journal of Chromatography 101: 414-416 (1974).

Mercier-Parot, L.: Disturbances in post-natal development of rats after maternal administration of cortisone during pregnancy or lactation. Comptes Rendus Hebdomadires des Seances de l'Academe des Sciences 240: 2259 (1955).

Mes, J.; Davies, D.J. and Miles, W.: Traces of mirex in some Canadian human milk samples. Bulletin of Environmental Contamination and Toxicology 19: 564-570 (1978).

Miller, G.E. and Stowe, C.M., Jr: Influence of oxytocin on diffusion of sulfonamides from plasma into bovine milk. Journal of Dairy Science 50: 840-846 (1967).

Miller, J.K. and Swanson, E.W.: Some factors affecting iodine secretion in milk. Journal of Dairy Science 46: 927-932 (1963).

Miller, G.E.; Banerjee, N.C. and Stowe, C.M., Jr: Diffusion of certain weak organic acids and bases across the bovine mammary gland membrane after systemic administration. Journal of Pharmacology and Experimental Therapeutics 157: 245-253 (1967a).

Miller, G.E.; Banerjee, N.C. and Stowe, C.M., Jr: Drug movement between bovine milk and plasma as affected by milk pH. Journal of Dairy Science 50: 1395-1403 (1967b).

Miller, G.E.; Peters, R.D.; Engebretsen, R.V. and Stowe, C.M.: Passage of pentobarbital and phenobarbital into bovine and caprine milk after systemic administration. Journal of Dairy Science 50: 769-772 (1967c).

Mills, E.S. and Topper, Y.J.: Some ultrastructural effects of insulin hydrocortisone and prolactin on mammary gland explants. Journal of Cell Biology 44: 310 (1970).

Mirkin, B.L.: Diphenylhydantoin: Placental transport, fetal localization, neonatal metabolism and potential teratogenic effect. Journal of Pediatrics 78: 329-337 (1971).

Mirkin, B.L.: (Ed.) Perinatal Pharmacology and Therapeutics, (Academic Press, New York 1976).

Morrison, S.D.: Human milk: Yield, proximate principles and inorganic constituents. Aberdeen, Scotland: Commonwealth Agricultural Bureau Technical Communication No. 18 (1952).

Mortimer, E.A., Jr: Drug toxicity from breast milk. Pediatrics 60: 780-781 (1977).

Morton, R.K.: Microsomal particles of normal cow's milk. Nature 171: 734-735 (1953).

Mulley, B.A.; Parr, G.D.; Pau, W.K.; Rye, R.M.; Mould, J.J. and Siddle, N.C.: Placental transfer of chlorthalidone and its elimination in maternal milk. European Journal of Clinical Pharmacology 13: 129-131 (1978).

Murthy, G.K. and Rhea, U.S.; Cadmium, copper, iron, lead, manganese and zinc in evaporated milk, infant products, and human milk. Journal of Dairy Science 54: 1001-1005 (1971).

Musial, C.J.; Hutzinger, O.; Zitko, V. and Crocker, J.: Presence of PCB, DDE, and DDT in human milk in the provinces of New Brunswick and Nova Scotia, Canada. Bulletin of Environmental Contamination and Toxicology 12: 258-267 (1974).

Neathery, M.W. and Miller, W.J.: Metabolism and toxicity of cadmium, mercury, and lead in animals: A review. Journal of Dairy Science 58: 1767-1781 (1975).

Nichols, B.L. and Nichols, V.N.: The biologic basis of lactation. Comprehensive Therapy 4: 63-70 (1979).

Nims, B.; Macy, I.G.; Hunscher, H. and Brown, M.: Variation in the composition of milk at four hour intervals during the day and night. American Journal of Diseases of Children 43: 828 (1932a).

Nims, B.; Macy, I.G.; Hunscher, H. and Brown, M.: Daily and monthly variations in milk components as observed in two successive lactation periods. American Journal of Diseases in Children 43: 1062 (1932b).

O'Brien, T.E.: Excretion of drugs in human milk. American Journal of Hospital Pharmacy 31: 844-854 (1974).

O'Brien, T.E.: Excretion of drugs in human milk. Nursing Digest, July/August 23-31 (1975).

Olszyna-Marzys, A.E.: Contaminants in human milk. Acta Paediatrica Scandinavica 67: 571-576 (1978).

Orme, M.L.'E.; Lewis, P.J.; de Swiet, M.; Serlin, M.J.; Sibeon, R.; Baty, J.D. and Breckenridge, A.M.: May mothers given warfarin breast-feed their infants? British Medical Journal 1: 1564-1565 (1977).

Overbach, A.M.: Part 3: Drugs that may cause fetal damage or cross into breast milk. R.N. 37 (Dec): 39-45 (1974).

Pacifici, G.M. and Placidi, G.F.: Rapid and sensitive electron-capture gas chromatographic method for the determination of pinazepam and its metabolites in human plasma, urine and milk. Journal of Chromatography 135: 133-139 (1977).

Panalaks, T.: A gas-chromatographic method for the determination of Vitamin D in fortified non-fat dried milk. Analyst 95: 862-867 (1970).

Parolaro, D.; Sala, M. and Gori, E.: Effect of intracerebroventricular administration of morphine upon intestinal motility in rats and its antagonism with naloxone. European Journal of Pharmacology 46: 329-338 (1977).

Patrick, M.J.; Tilstone, W.J. and Reavey, P.: Diazepam and breast-feeding. Lancet 1: 542-543 (1972).

Peaker, M.: Lactation: Some cardiovascular and metabolic consequences, and the mechanisms of lactose and ion secretion into milk. Ciba Foundation Symposium 45: 87-101 (1976).

Peeters, G.; Coussens, R. and Sierens, G.: Physiology of the nerves in the bovine mammary gland. Archives Internationales de Pharmacodynamie et de Therapie 79: 75-82 (1949).

Pendleton, R.C. and Lloyd, R.D.: Forecasting ^{137}Cs in humans resulting from ^{137}Cs in reactor effluents. Health Physics 26: 351-358 (1974).

Perlman, H.H.; Dannenberg, A.M. and Sokofoff, N.: The excretion of nicotine in breast milk and urine from cigarette smoking. Journal of the American Medical Association 120: 1003-1009 (1942).

Pesendorfer, H.: Ruckstande von Organochlorpestiziden (DDT u.a.) und Polychlorierten Biphenylen

(PCB's) in der Mutter Milch. Wiener Klinische Wochenschrift 87: 732-736 (1975).

Pfielsticker, K.: Pesticide in der Kinderernhrung. Monatsschrift fur Kinderheilkunde 121: 551-553 (1973).

Picciano, M.F. and Guthrie, H.A.: Copper, iron and zinc contents of mature human milk. American Journal of Clinical Nutrition 29: 242 (1976).

Picciano, F.; Guthrie, H.A. and Sheehe, D.M.: The cholesterol content of human milk. Clinical Pediatrics 17: 359-362 (1978).

Pickles, V.R.: Blood flow estimations as indices of mammary activity. Journal of Obstetrics and Gynaecology of the British Commonwealth 60: 301-311 (1953).

Piper, D.W. and Fenton, B.: pH stability and activity curves of pepsin with special reference to their clinical importance. Gut 6: 506-508 (1965).

Posner, A.C. et al.: Tetracycline in obstetric infections. Antibiotics Annual 1955-1956, p.345 (American Society for Microbiology, Ann Arbor 1956).

Potter, J.M. and Nestel, R.J.: The effect of dietary fatty acids and cholesterol on the milk lipids of lactating women and the plasma cholesterol of breast fed infants. American Journal of Clinical Nutrition 29: 54 (1976).

Pynnonen, S. and Sillanpaa, M.: Carbamazepine and mother's milk. Lancet 2: 563 (1975).

Pynnonen, S.; Kanto, J.; Sillanpaa, M. and Erkkola, R.: Carbamazepine: Placental transport, tissue concentrations in foetus and newborn, and level in milk. Acta Pharmacology and Toxicology 41: 244-253 (1977).

Quinby, G.E.; Armstrong, J.F. and Durham, W.F.: DDT in human milk. Nature 207: 726-728 (1965).

Rainbow, K.A.: Magnesium sulfate and breast milk. Journal of the American Medical Association 146: 298 (1951).

Rane, A.: Clinical pharmacokinetics of antiepileptic drugs in children. Pharmacology and Therapeutics C2: 251-267 (1978).

Rane, A.; Garle, M. and Sjoqvist, F.: Plasma disappearance of transplacentally transferred diphenylhydantoin in the newborn studied by mass fragmentography. Clinical Pharmacology and Therapeutics 15: 39-49 (1974).

Rasmussen, F.: Mammary excretion of sulphonamides. Acta Pharmacologica et Toxicologica 15: 139-148 (1958).

Rasmussen, F.: Mammary excretion of benzylpenicillin, erythromycin, and penethamate hydroiodide. Acta Pharmacologica et Toxicologica 16: 194-200 (1959).

Rasmussen, F.: Mammary excretion of antipyrine, ethanol, and urea. Acta Veterinaria Scandinavica 2: 151-156 (1961).

Rasmussen, F.: The mammary blood flow in the goat as measured by antipyrine absorption. Acta Veterinaria Scandinavica 4: 271-280 (1963).

Rasmussen, F.: The mammary blood flow in the cow as measured by the antipyrine absorption method. Acta Veterinaria Scandinavica 6: 135-149 (1965).

Rasmussen, F.: Studies on the Mammary Excretion and Absorption of Drugs (Mortensen, Copenhagen 1966).

Rasmussen, F.: Mammary excretion of lincomycin in cows. Acta Veterinaria Scandinavica 7: 97-98 (1966a).

Rasmussen, F.: Active mammary excretion of N[4]-acetylated p-aminohippuri acid. Acta Veterinaria Scandinavica 10: 193-194 (1969a).

Rasmussen, F.: Active mammary excretion of N[4]-acetylated sulphanilamide. Acta Veterinaria Scandinavica 10: 402-403 (1969b).

Rasmussen, F.: Excretion of drugs by milk; in Brodie and Gillette (Eds) Concepts in Biochemical Pharmacology (Springer-Verlag, Berlin, Heidelberg, New York 1971).

Rasmussen, F.: The mechanism of drug secretion into milk; in Galli (Ed.) Dietary Lipids and Postnatal Development, pp.231-245 (Raven Press, New York 1973).

Rasmussen, F. and Linzell, J.L.: The accuracy of the indicator absorption method of measuring mammary blood flow by the Fick principle. Quarterly Journal of Experimental Physiology 49: 219-225 (1964).

Rasmussen, F. and Linzell, J.L.: The acetylation of sulphanilamide by mammary tissue of lactating goats. Biochemical Pharmacology 16: 918-919 (1967).

Read, W.W.C.; Lutz, P.G. and Tashjian, A.: Human milk lipids. II. The influence of dietary carbohydrates and fat on the fatty acids of mature milk. A study in four ethnic groups. American Journal of Clinical Nutrition 17: 180 (1965).

Read, W.W.C. and Sarrif, A.: Human milk lipids. I. Changes in fatty acid composition of early colostrum. American Journal of Clinical Nutrition 17: 177 (1965).

Rees, J.A.; Glass, R.C. and Sporne, G.A.: Serum and breast milk concentrations of dothiepin. Practitioner 217: 686 (1976).

Reineke, E.P.: Factors affecting the secretion of iodine into milk of lactating goats. Journal of Dairy Science 44: 937-942 (1961).

Resman, B.H.; Blumenthal, H.P. and Jusko, W.J.: Breast milk distribution of theobromine from chocolate. Journal of Pediatrics 91: 477-480 (1977).

Reynolds, M.: Relationship of mammary circulation and oxygen consumption to lactogenesis; in Lactogenesis, the Initiation of Milk Secretion at Parturition (University of Pennsylvania Press, Philadelphia 1969).

Reynolds, M.; Linzell, J.L. and Rasmussen, F.: Comparison of four methods for measuring mammary blood flow in conscious goats. American Journal of Physiology 214: 1415-1424 (1968).

Rhodin, J.A.G.: An Atlas of Histology (Oxford University Press, New York 1975).

Risebrough, R.W.: In report of the Secretary's Commission of pesticides and their relationship to environmental health, U.S. Department of Health, Education and Welfare, p.258 (1969).

Rivera, E.M. and Bern, H.A.: Influence of insulin on maintenance and secretory stimulation of mouse mammary tissues by hormones in organ culture. Endocrinology 69: 340-353 (1961).

Ryan, J.J.; Lee, Y.C. Dupont, J.A. and Charbonneau, C.F.: A screening method for determining nitrofuran drug residues in animal tissues. Journal of the Association of Official Analytical Chemists 58: 1227-1231 (1975).

Sack, J.; Amado, O. and Lunenfeld, B.: Thyroxine concentration in human milk. Journal of Clinical Endocrinology and Metabolism 45: 171-173 (1977).

St. John, L.E. and Lisk, D.J.: A feeding study with the herbicide, Kerb [N(1,1-dimethylpropynyl)-3,5-dichlorobenzamide] in the dairy cow. Bulletin of Environmental Contamination and Toxicology 13: 433-435 (1975).

Sauerhoff, M.W. and Michaelson, I.A.: Hyperactivity and brain catecholamines in lead-exposed developing rats. Science 182: 1022-1024 (1973).

Savage, E.P.; Tessari, J.D.; Malberg, J.W.; Wheeler, H.W. and Bagby, J.R.: A search for polychlorinated biphenyls in human milk in rural Colorado. Bulletin of Environmental Contamination and Toxicology 9: 222-226 (1973).

Schanker, L.S.: Passage of drugs across body membranes. Pharmacological Reviews 14: 501-530 (1962).

Schanker, L.S.: Absorption of drugs from the gastrointestinal tract; in Brodie and Gillette (Eds) Handbook of Experimental Pharmacology, Vol. XXVIII, pp.9-24 (Springer-Verlag, Berlin, Heidelberg, New York 1971).

Schilf, E. and Wohinz, R.: Uber das Vorkommen von Coffein in der Frauenmilch nach GenuB von Kaffee. Archiv fuer Gynaekologie 134: 201-204 (1928).

Schou, M. and Amdisen, A.: Lithium and pregnancy. III. Lithium ingestion by children breast-fed by women on lithium treatment. British Medical Journal 2: 138 (1973).

Schroeder, H.A. and Nason, A.P.: Trace-element analysis. Clinical Chemistry 17: 461-474 (1971).

Schulte-Lobbert, F.S. and Bohm, G.: Determination of cadmium in human milk during lactation. Archives of Toxicology 37: 155-157 (1977).

Schumacher, H.M.: Uber Coffeinausscheidung in die Frauenmilch. Medizinische Welt 10: 408-411 (1936).

Sedgwick, J.P.: A preliminary report of the study of breast-feeding in Minneapolis. American Journal of Diseases of Children 21: 455 (1921).

Shani (Mishkinsky), J.; Ziv, G.; Givant, Y.; Buchman, O. and Sulman, F.G.: Pharmacokinetic studies of triated perphenazine: Passage from blood to milk in cows and ewes. Archives Internationales de Pharmacodynamie et de Therapie 207: 44-56 (1974).

Shimada, T. and Ugawa, M.: Induction of liver microsomal drug metabolism by polychlorinated biphenyls whose gas chromatographic profile having much in common with that in human milk. Bulletin of Environmental Contamination Toxicology 19: 198-205 (1978).

Shirkey, H.: Drug excretion in breast milk; in Avery (Ed) Drug Treatment 2nd ed. pp.113-116 (ADIS Press, Sydney and New York: Churchill Livingstone, Edinburgh 1980).

Sidman, M.: Behavioral pharmacology. Psychopharmacologia 1: 1-19 (1959).

Sidman, M.: Tactics of Scientific Research (Basic Books, New York, 1960).

Singer, S.J.: Architecture and topography of biologic membranes. Hospital Practice 8: 81-90 (1973).

Siyali, D.S.: Polychlorinated biphenyls, hexachlorobenzene and other organochlorine pesticides in human milk. Medical Journal of Australia 2: 815-818 (1973).

Smadel, J.E.; Woodward, T.E.; Ley, H.L., Jr. and Lewthwaite, R.: Chloramphenicol (chloromycetin) in the treatment of tsutsugamushi disease (scrub typhus). Journal of Clinical Investigation 28: 1196-1215 (1949).

Smals, A.G.; Kloppenborg, P.W.; Njo, K.T.; Knoben, J.M. and Ruland, G.M.: Alcohol induced cushingoid syndrome. British Medical Journal 2: 1298 (1976).

Snowdon, C.T.: Learning deficits in lead-injected rats. Pharmacology, Biochemistry and Behavior 1: 599-603 (1973).

Sollmann, T.: A Manual of Pharmacology, 8th Ed. (W.B. Saunders, Philadelphia 1957).

Somogyi, A. and Gugler, R.: Cimetidine excretion into breast milk. British Journal of Clinical Pharmacology 7: 627-629 (1979).

Stechler, G.: Newborn attention as affected by medication during labor. Science 144: 315-317 (1964).

Stewart, J.C. and Vidor, G.I.: Thyrotoxicosis induced by iodine contamination of foods — a common unrecognized condition? British Medical Journal 1: 372-375 (1976).

Stewart, J.J.; Weisbrodt, N.W. and Burks, T.F.: Central and peripheral actions of morphine on intestinal transit. Journal of Pharmacology and Experimental Therapeutics 205: 547-555 (1978).

Stewart, W.C. and Sinclair, R.G.: The absence of ricinoleic acid from phospholipids of rats fed castor oil. Archives of Biochemistry 8: 7-11 (1945).

Street, J.C.: DDT antagonism to dieldrin storage in adipose tissue of rats. Science 146: 1580-1581 (1964).

Street, J.C.; Wang, M. and Blau, A.D.: Drug effects on dieldrin storage in rat tissue. Bulletin of Environmental Contamination and Toxicology 1: 6-15 (1966).

Sturman, J.A.; Gaull, G. and Raiha, N.C.R.: Absence of cystathionase in human fetal liver: is cystine essential? Science 169: 74-76 (1970).

Svanberg, V.; Gebre-Mehden, U.; Ljungqvist, B. and Olsson, M.: Breast milk composition in Ethiopian and Swedish mothers. III. Aminoacids and other nitrogenous substances. American Journal of Clinical Nutrition 30: 499 (1977).

Svensmark, A.; Schiller, P.I. and Buchthal, F.: 5,5-diphenylhydantoin (Dilantin) blood levels after oral or intravenous dosage in men. Acta Pharmacologica et Toxicologica 16: 331-346 (1960).

Sykes, P.A. and Quarrie, J.: Lithium carbonate and breast feeding. British Medical Journal 2: 1299 (1976).

Taitz, L.S.: Modification of weight gain by dietary changes in a population of Sheffield neonates. Archives of Disease in Childhood 50: 746 (1975).

Takyi, B.E.: Excretion of drugs in human milk. Journal of Hospital Pharmacy 28: 317-326 (1970).

Tarjan, R.; Kramer, M.; Szoke, K. et al.: The effect of different factors on the composition of human milk.

II. The composition of human milk during lactation. Nutritio et Dieta 7: 136 (1965).

Terwilliger, W.G. and Hatcher, R.A.: Morphine and quinine in human milk. Surgery, Gynecology and Obstetrics 58: 823-826 (1934).

Thomas, L.: The Medusa and the Snail (Viking Press, New York 1979).

Thomas, M.J.; Danutra, V.; Read, G.F.; Hillier, S.G. and Griffiths, K.: The detection and measurement of D-norgestrel in human milk using Sephadex LH 20 chromatography and radioimmunoassay. Steroids 30: 349-361 (1977).

Thompson, R.D.; Nagasawa, H.T. and Jenne, J.W.: Determination of theophylline and its metabolites in human urine and serum by high-pressure liquid chromatography. Journal of Laboratory and Clinical Medicine 84: 584-593 (1974).

Tunnessen, W.W. and Hertz, G.C.: Toxic effects of lithium in newborn infants: A commentary. Journal of Pediatrics 81: 804-807 (1972).

Turkington, R.W.; Majumder, G.C. and Riddle, M.: Inhibition of mammary gland differentiation in vitro by 5-bromo-2'-deoxyuridine. Journal of Biological Chemistry 246: 1814 (1971).

Tyson, R.M.; Shrader, E.A. and Perlman, H.H.: Drugs transmitted through breast milk. Part II. Journal of Pediatrics 13: 86-90 (1938).

Tyson, R.M.; Shrader, E.A. and Perlman, H.H.: Drugs transmitted through breast milk. Part II? Journal of Pediatrics 13: 86-90 (1938).

Unna, K.R.; Glaser, K.; Lipton, E. and Patterson, P.R.: Dosage of drugs in infants and children. I. Atropine. Pediatrics (Springfield) 6: 197-207 (1950).

Vahlquist, B.: Evolution of breast feeding in Europe. Journal of Tropical Pediatrics 21: 11 (1975).

van As, A.: Beta-adrenergic stimulant bronchodilators; in Stein (Ed) New Directions in Asthma, pp.415-431 (American College of Chest Physicians, Park Ridge, Illinois 1975).

van Os, F.H.L.: Anthraquinone derivatives in vegetable laxatives. Pharmacology 14 (Suppl. 1): 7-17 (1976).

van Os, F.H.L.: Some aspects of the pharmacology of anthraquinone drugs. Pharmacology 14 (Suppl. 1): 18-29 (1976a).

Varsano, I.; Fischl, J. and Shochet, S.B.: The excretion of orally ingested nitrofurantoin in human milk. Journal of Pediatrics 82: 886-887 (1973).

Vorherr, H.: To breast-feed or not to breast-feed? Postgraduate Medicine 51: 127-134 (1972).

Vorherr, H.: The Breast Morphology, Physiology and Lactation (Academic Press, New York, San Francisco, London 1974a).

Vorherr, H.: Drug excretion in breast milk. Postgraduate Medicine 56: 97-104 (1974b).

Voshioka, H.; Cho, K.; Takinoto, M.; Naruyana, S. and Shimizu, T.: Transfer of cefazolin into human milk. Journal of Pediatrics 94: 151-152 (1979).

Vuori, E.; Tyllinen, H.; Kuitunen, P. and Paganus, A.: The occurrence and origin of DDT in human milk. Acta Paediatrica Scandinavica 66: 761-765 (1977).

Wagner, G. and Fuchs, A.R.: Effect of ethanol on uterine activity during suckling in post-partum women. Acta Endocrinologica 58: 133-141 (1968).

Wagner, J.G.; Northam, J.I.; Alway, C.D. and Carpenter, O.S.: Blood levels of drug at the equilibrium state after multiple dosing. Nature 207: 1391-1402 (1969).

Waletzky, L.R. and Herman, E.C.: Relactation. American Family Physician 14: 69 (1976).

Walgren, A.: Breast milk consumption of healthy full-term infants. Acta Paediatrica 32: 778 (1945).

Waller, H.: The early failure of breast feeding. A clinical study of its causes and their prevention. Archives of Disease in Childhood 21: 1-12 (1946).

Watkins, W.M. and Hassid, W.Z.: Synthesis of lactose by particulate enzyme preparations from guinea pig and bovine mammary glands. Journal of Biological Chemistry 237: 1432-1440 (1962).

Watson, W.C. and Gordon, R.S.: Studies on the digestion, absorption and metabolism of castor oil. Biochemical Pharmacology 11: 229-236 (1962).

Watson, W.C.; Gordon, R.S.; Karmen, A. and Jover, A.: The absorption and excretion of castor oil in man. Journal of Pharmacy and Pharmacology 15: 183-188 (1963).

Wegner, T.N.: Simple and sensitive procedure for determining nitrate and nitrite in mixtures in biological fluids. Journal of Dairy Science 55: 642-644 (1972).

Weinstein, M.R. and Goldfield, M.: Lithium carbonate treatment during pregnancy. Diseases of the Nervous System 30: 823-832 (1969).

Weiss, B. and Laties, V.G. (Eds) Behavioral Toxicology (Plenum Press, New York, 1975).

Welby, M.; O'Halloran, M.W. and Wellby, M.L.: Maternal diet and lipid composition of breast milk. Lancet 2: 458 (1973).

Werthmann, M.W. and Krees, S.V.: Excretion of chlorothiazine in human breast milk. Journal of Pediatrics 81: 781-783 (1972).

West, R.W.; Wilson, D.J. and Schaffner, W.: Hexachlorophene concentrations in human milk. Bulletin of Environmental Contamination and Toxicology 13: 167-169 (1975).

Wichelow, M.G.: Success and failure in relation to energy intake. Proceedings of the Nutrition Society 35: 62A (1976).

Williams, R.H.; Kay, G.A. and Jandorf, B.J.: Thiouracil: its absorption, distribution, and excretion. Journal of Clinical Investigation 23: 613-627 (1944).

White, M.: Breast feeding and drugs in human milk. La Leche League International, Inc., pp.1-31 (Franklin Park, Illinois 1978).

Widdowson, E.M.; Southgate, D.A.T. and Schutz, Y.: Comparison of dried milk preparations for babies on sale in 7 European countries. I. Protein, fat, carbohydrate and inorganic constituents. Archives of Disease in Childhood 49: 867-873 (1974).

Wilson, D.J.; Locker, D.J.; Ritzen, C.A.; Watson, J.T. and Schaffner, W.: DDT concentrations in human milk. American Journal of Diseases of Children 125: 814-817 (1973).

Wilson, H.T.: Intestinal Absorption (W.B. Saunders, Philadelphia 1962).

Wilson, J.T.: Pragmatic assessment of medicines available for young children and pregnant or breast-feeding women; in Morselli, Garattini and Serini (Eds) Basic and Therapeutic Aspects of Perinatal Pharmacology, pp.411-421 (Raven Press, New York 1975).

Winter, M.; Thomas, M.; Wernick, S.; Levin, S. and Farvar, M.T.: Analysis of pesticide residues in 290 samples of Guatemalan mothers' milk. Bulletin of Environmental Contamination and Toxicology 16: 652-657 (1976).

Wiskerchen, J.E. and Weishaar, J.: Quantitative determination of chlorobutanol in milk by gas-liquid chromatography. Journal of the Association of Official Analytical Chemists 55: 948-950 (1972).

Woodard, B.T.; Ferguson, B.B. and Wilson, D.J.: DDT levels in milk of rural indigent blacks. American Journal of Diseases of Children 130: 400-403 (1976).

Yurchak, A.M. and Jusko, W.J.: Theophylline secretion into breast milk. Pediatrics 57: 518-520 (1976).

Ziv, G.; Shani (Mishkinsky), J.; Givant, Y.; Buchman, O. and Sulman, F.G.: Distribution of tritiated haloperidol in lactating and pregnant cows and ewes. Archives Internationales de Pharmacodynamie et Therapie 212: 154-163 (1974).

Appendix

Some synonyms and proprietary names of drugs and chemicals mentioned.

Drug	Synonym	Proprietary name(s)
Adrenaline	Epinephrine	
Aminophyllline	Theophylline and ethylenediamine	
Amitriptyline		'Triptizol'
Bendrofluazide	Bendroflumethiazide	'Neo-Naclex' 'Naturetin'
Bisacodyl		'Dulcolax' 'Bicol' 'Biscolax'
Butabarbitone	Secbutobarbitone, butabarbital	
Carbamazepine		'Tegretol'
Casanthrol		'Peristim Forte'
Chloramphenicol		'Chloromycetin'
Chlorbutol	Chlorobutanol, chlorbutanol	

Drug	Synonym	Proprietary name(s)
Chlordiazepoxide		'Librium'
Chlorothiazide		'Saluric'
		'Chlotride'
Chlorpromazine		'Largactil'
Chlorthalidone	Chlortalidone	'Hygroton'
Cimetidine		'Tagamet'
Clindamycin		'Dalacin C'
Clorazepate		'Tranxene'
Danthron	Dianthron	'Dorbanex'
DDE	1,1-Dichloro-2 2 bis (p-chlorophenyl)ethylene	
Dexbrompheniramine brompheniramine		'Disomer'
Diazepam		'Valium'
Dicophane	Chlorophenothane, DDT, 1,1-trichloro-2-2 bis (p-chlorophenyl)ethane	
Dicoumarol	Dicumarol	
Diphenhydramine		'Benadryl'
Diphenoxylate		'Lomotil'
Dothiepin	Dosulepin, prothiadene	'Prothiaden'
Erythromycin		'Erythrocin', 'Ilosene', 'Ilotycin'
Ethyl Biscoumacetate	Ethyldicoumarol	'Tromexan'
Fenoterol		'Berotec'
Flufenamic acid		'Arlef'
Frusemide	Furosemide	'Lasix'
Gamma benzene hexachloride	Gamma-BHC, lindane	'Lorexane'
Glutethimide		'Doriden'
Glycopyrrolate	Glycopyrronium	'Robinul'
Guanethidine		'Ismelin'
Haloperidol		'Serenace'
Halothane		'Fluothane'
Heptabarbitone	Heptabarbital	'Medomin'
Hexachlorobenzene	HCB	
Hydrallazine	Hydralazine, apressinum	'Apresoline'

Drug	Synonym	Proprietary name(s)
Imipramine		'Tofranil'
Isoetharine	Isopropylethylnoradrenaline	'Numotac'
Isoprenaline	Isoproterenol	'Aleudrin'
Isopropamide		'Tyrimide'
Lignocaine	Lidocaine	'Xylocaine'
Lincomyin		'Lincocin'
Loperamide		'Imodium'
Mefanamic acid		'Ponstan'
Mepenzolate		'Cantil'
Methadone	Amidone, phenadone	'Physeptone'
Methotrexate	Amethopterin	
Methylglyoxal	Mitoguazone	'Methyl-GAG'
Methylphenidate	Methyl phenidate	'Ritalin'
Mitotane	DDD,	
	1,1-dichloro-2 2-bis	'Lysodren'
	(p-chlorophenyl)ethane	
Nitrofurantoin		'Furadantin'
Norgestrel		'Neogest',
Nortriplyline		'Allegron',
		'Aventyl',
Orciprenaline	Metaproterenol	'Alupent',
		'Metaprel',
Oxazepam		'Serenid'
Oxyphenonium		'Antrenyl'
Penethamate hydriodide	Diethyaminoethyl penicillin	'Bronchocilline',
	G hydroiodide	'Leocillin'
Pentobarbitone	Pentobarbital	
Perphenazine		'Fentazin'
		'Trilafon'
Phenazone	Antipyrine	
Phenobarbitone	Phenobarbital	
Phenlybutazone		'Butazolidin'
Phenytoin	Diphenylhydantoin	'Epanutin',
		'Dilantin',
		'Garoin'
Pinazepam		'Domar'
Prochlorperazine	Prochlorpemazine	'Stemetil',
		'Vertigon'
Propantheline		'Pro-Banthine'
Propranolol		'Inderal'

Drug	Synonym	Proprietary names(s)
Pseudoephedrine	*d*-Isoephedrine	
Pyrimethamine		'Daraprim'
Quinalbarbitone	Secobarbital	'Seconal'
Reserpine		'Serpasil'
Salbutamol	Albuterol	'Ventolin', 'Sultanol'
Sulfadoxine	Sulphormethoxine	'Fanasil'
Sulphadimidine	Sulfamethazine	
Terbutaline		'Bricanyl', 'Brethine'
Thiopentone	Thiopental	'Pentothal', 'Intraval'
Tolbutamide		'Rastinon', 'Orinase', 'Oribetic'
Trifluoperazine		'Stelabid'
Tripelennamine		'Pyribenzamine'
Trimeprazine		'Vallergan'

Subject Index